Jiro Suzuki

Moyamoya Disease

With 145 Figures

Springer-Verlag
Berlin Heidelberg New York Tokyo

Professor JIRO SUZUKI, M. D.
Tohoku University School of Medicine
Institute of Brain Diseases
Division of Neurosurgery
2-1 Seiryo-Cho, Sendai 980, Japan

Translation of: Moyamoya Byō

ISBN-13: 978-3-540-15778-6 e-ISBN-13: 978-3-642-95483-2
DOI: 10.1007/978-3-642-95483-2

Library of Congress Cataloging-in-Publication Data. Suzuki, Jiro, 1924– Moyamoya disease. Translation of: Moyamoya byō. Bibliography: p. Includes index. 1. Moyamoya disease. I. Title. [DNLM: 1. Arterial Occlusive Diseases. WG510 S968m] RC388.5.S8813 1986 616.1'3 85-26118

Typesetting: fotosatz & design, Berchtesgaden

2125/3130-543210

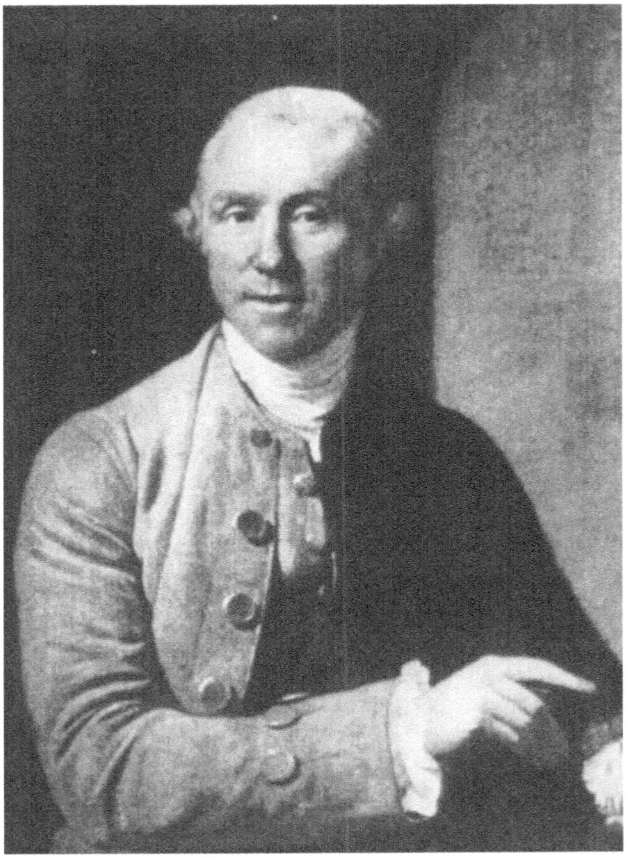

JOHN HUNTER (1728–1793)

"Blood goes where it is needed," he said in 1785

Moyamoya vessels are collateral pathways of the brain
JIRO SUZUKI (1963)

Preface

The first mention of moyamoya disease as a distinct disease entity was in a paper I published in 1965. The abnormal net-like vessels at the base of the brain seen in cerebral angiograms of this disease were described by most native speakers of Japanese as "moyamoya," a Japanese expression for something hazy, such as a puff of cigarette smoke drifting in the air. In fact, prior to my advocacy of this term, this type of vascular network was often referred to as "moyamoya vessels" by Japanese researchers.

In 1969, Dr. A. Takaku and I submitted a paper to the *Archives of Neurology* entitled "A Disease Showing Abnormal Net-like Vessels at the base of the Brain," with a subtitle of "Moyamoya Disease." The editor, however, interchanged the main title and the subtitle and brought this term "moyamoya" to fame! Since then, researchers throughout the world have been using this poetic word! For a nicknaming godfather like me, it is a special joy to have this Japanese word enter the honored ranks of medical terminology.

My first publication concerning this lesion was a report discussing six cases in 1963. Therefore it is now 20 years since I first became aware of and started to study moyamoya disease. At first, I merely thought that it was a strange vascular network, unique to these first few patients, and I reported these cases as being cases of acquired collateral vessels. Thereafter, many researchers speculated that it might be a form of vascular tumor, and intense debate as to whether this disease is congenital or acquired began. Currently, it is generally thought that moyamoya vessels are collateral pathways formed due to gradually progressing stenosis of the terminal portion of the internal carotid artery, for reasons unknown.

Although the incidence of moyamoya disease is still said to be higher in Japan than elsewhere, in recent years there have been reports of cases from both the East and the West, and moyamoya disease has become a matter of great interest to researchers throughout the world.

Through the combined efforts of many researchers over the past 2 decades, many aspects of moyamoya disease have been clarified. These include the incidence according to age and sex, symptomatology, angiographical characteristics, electroencephalographical characteristics, and details of the cerebral blood flow in such cases. This is not to say, however, that unresolved problems no longer exist. Most importantly, it is still unclear what causal factors are involved in the progressive narrowing and occlusion of the terminal portion of the internal carotid artery bilaterally. Since the vascular abnormalities at this portion are the essence of the disease, it is apparent that some fundamental questions still need to be answered.

Nevertheless, as readers of this volume will understand, our systemic autopsy studies and animal research have suggested that moyamoya disease may be caused by immunological arteritis throughout the body, which manifests itself most easily and most severely at those cerebral arteries which receive innervation from the superior cervical sympathetic ganglia.

Having actively researched this disease for 20 years, we, the Sendai Group of Neurosurgeons, decided to summarize our experiences and research in a single volume. With each of the researchers reporting on his own research interests related to moyamoya disease, we hav tried to cover all aspects of this disease, including its etiology.

I am hopeful that this volume will serve as an introduction and an up-to-date summary of our current knowledge concerning moyamoya disease for physicians and researchers throughout the world.

I would like to express my thanks to all my colleagues and to the nurses and paramedical staff for their untiring efforts during this period. I also acknowledge, with thanks, the valuable assistance of Mr. Norman D. Cook in improving the English throughout the book. Finally, I must say that this publication has been made possible by the enthusiasm and efforts of the various doctors (T. Wada, N. Kodama, T. Kayama, H. Niizuma, H. Ohyama, T. Yoshimoto, A. Ogawa, N. Nakamura, Y. Sakurai, S. Komatsu, S. Kanayama, Y. Nagamine, T. Onuma, N. Kasai, T. Yonemitsu, T. Watanabe, M. Suzuki, R. Katakura and A. Takahashi) in our department, and especially Drs. S. Fujiwara, H. Seki and M. Kameyama.

JIRO SUZUKI

Contents

1 History and Definition

Characteristically, cerebral angiograms in cases of moyamoya disease show stenosis or occlusion of the terminal portion of the internal carotid artery bilaterally. Moreover, in the vicinity of the base of the brain, abnormal net-like vessels can also often be seen bilaterally, showing differences in the degree of the vascular network on the left and right. Depending upon the individual case, angiographical abnormalities are seen in the defects of the middle and/or anterior cerebral arteries, and sometimes of all the main cerebral arteries including the posterior cerebral artery (Fig. 1).

Due to the efforts of many researches over the past 2 decades, it has become possible to make a nearly certain diagnosis of moyamoya disease based solely upon clinical symptoms and electroencephalographic findings, but an exact diagnosis must ultimately rely upon cerebral angiography.

Although the incidence of this disease has been particularly high among the Japanese and research reports from Japan are numerous, in recent years cases have been reported throughout the world, indicating that moyamoya disease is not limited to certain races or nationalities. It is now widely held that moyamoya vessels are collateral pathways brought about by slowly progressing vascular stenosis at the bilateral terminal portions of the internal carotid artery; the causal factors are as yet unknown.

The first cerebral angiograms of this disease were reported in 1955 at the 14th Meeting of the Japan Neurosurgical Society by Shimizu and Takeuchi [267]. These findings were reported as hypoplasia of the bilateral internal carotid arteries and were later published as a case report by Takeuchi in 1957 [314]. Thereafter, there sporadically appeared reports of angiograms, now understood to be suggestive of moyamoya disease, but in all such cases the angiograms were interpreted as showing congenital anomalies or vascular tumor [2, 99, 150, 153, 167, 184, 209, 213, 214, 258]. In 1957, Kudo reported a case of hypoplasia of the circle of Willis, again interpreted as a congenital vascular anomaly [150].

At the 22nd Meeting of the Japan Neurosurgical Society in 1963, Suzuki et al. [288] reported various findings on six cases, which we had experienced until then. We maintained that such abnormal net-like vessels at the base of the brain were collateral pathways formed due to acquired, gradual stenosis of the terminal portion of the internal carotid artery and constituted a single clinical entity. Our interpretation was severely criticized by several researchers at the time. During the same year, Moriyasu [184] reported that similar cases could be found among patients with apoplexy.

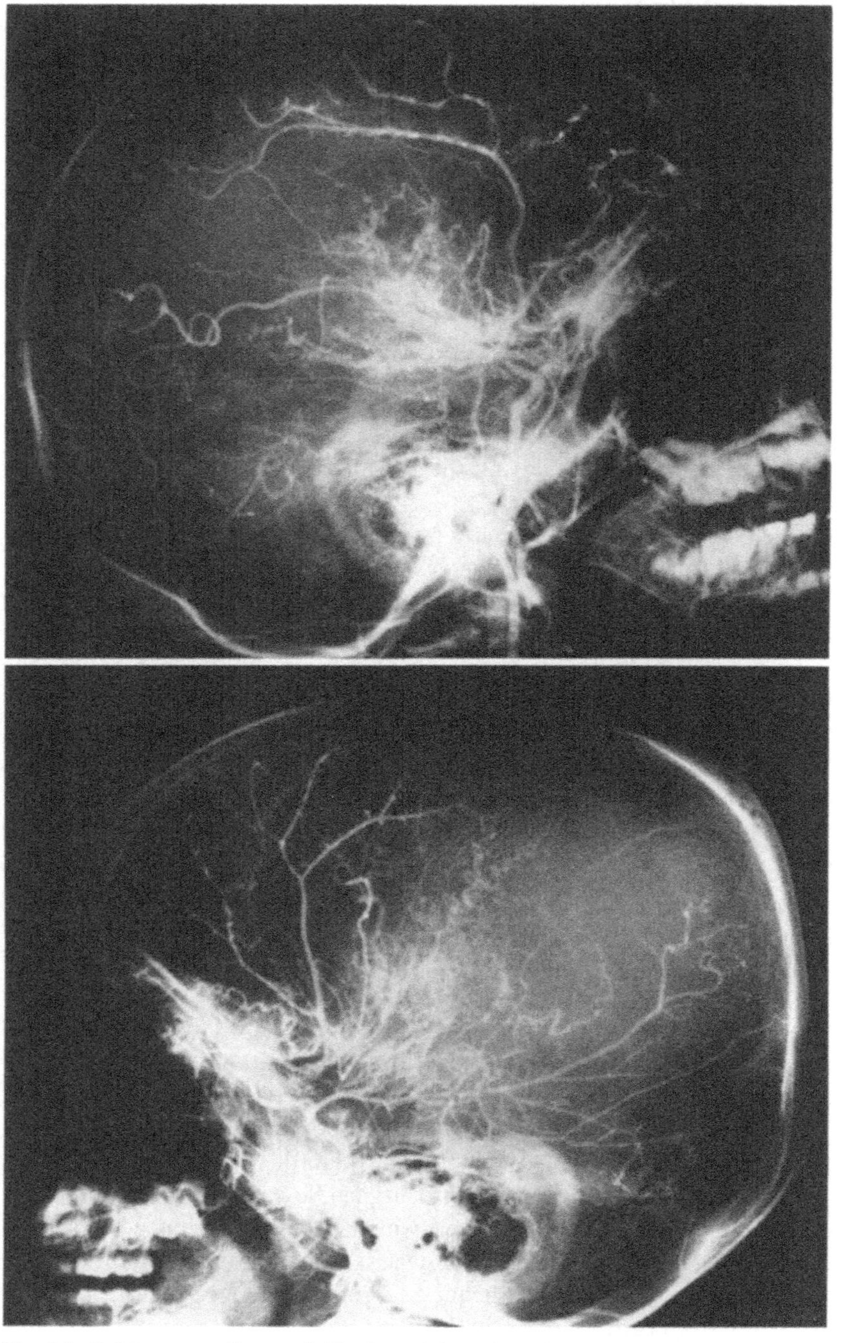

A

B

Fig. 1 A, B. Moyamoya disease. **A** The lateral view of the right carotid angiogram of a 2-year-old girl. **B** The lateral view of the left carotid angiogram of the same case at 4 years old. These photographs show narrowings at the terminal portions of bilateral internal carotid arteries and typical moyamoya vessels at the base of the brain (basal moyamoya, see Chap. 3)

During the following year many researchers in Japan reported such cases [43, 46, 65, 94, 305, 308, 332]. The first such report outside of Japan was made by W. Weidner et al. [342] in 1965 — a case of an American woman of Japanese descent. In the same year, Krayenbühl and Yasargil [141] published the cerebral angiograms of one such case in Krayenbühl's textbook, noted that such cerebral vessels were an extremely rare anomaly, and labeled the condition *Kapillare diffuse cerebrale Angioectasie.*

Also in 1965 Leeds and Abbott [160] reported two such cases, and in 1967 Gerlach et al. [49] reported a similar case. Since then the number of reports of moyamoya disease from the West has gradually increased [17, 21, 22, 27, 29, 31, 38, 47, 48, 57, 58, 77, 89, 91, 126, 140, 158, 161–163, 182, 186, 222, 235, 240, 252, 255, 262, 268, 326, 337, 338, 339, 359, 360], and it is now clear that this disease is not restricted to certain racial genotypes or localities. In Japan, analysis of a large number of cases of moyamoya disease and basic research on this disease have progressed rapidly [146, 151, 214, 216, 208, 289, 290].

In 1977, the Japanese government recommended research into the epidemiology, clinical symptomatology, pathophysiology, causal genesis, and treatment of moyamoya disease and consequently organized a research group for that purpose.

As is apparent from these facts, research on moyamoya disease in Japan has become rather intense over the past 20 years, and by the end of 1982 more than 2000 cases had been reported. The overall clinical picture of this disease has therefore come into focus. It must be said, however, that problems concerning etiology and treatment remain, and the question as to why there appear to be relatively more cases in Japan is yet unanswered.

A surprisingly large variety of labels for this condition have been suggested. These labels include: occlusive disease of the circle of Willis [143], cerebral juxtabasal teleangiectasia [11, 258, 259], hemiangiomatous malformation of the bilateral internal carotid arteries at the base of the brain [209], cerebral arterial rete [60], and Nishimoto's disease [211].

In 1965, the author suggested the name »moyamoya disease« in two published papers [290, 291]. »Moyamoya« was thought to be appropriate since the abnormal net-like vessels at the base of the brain, as seen in angiograms, are hazy in appearance — like a puff of cigarette smoke drifting in the air, which is commonly described as »moyamoya« by native speakers of Japanese. As described below, moreover, in follow-up angiograms of this disease in young patients, the sequential changes — from an initially thick »cloud,« to a gradually thinning and shrinking »fog,« to the eventual disappearance of the net-like vessels around the internal carotid artery — are also reminiscent of the misty »moyamoya« changes in cigarette smoke.

Certainly, »moyamoya« is an unusual word to enter into medical terminology, but it is appropriate for a number of reasons. It expresses the fact that its etiology is as hazy as the pattern of the abnormal vessels itself. Moreover, the disease was first reported in Japan and continues to show a high incidence there. Usage of a

Japanese word emphasizes these facts and has thus far been well received in the West as well as in Japan. Since the publication of the paper entitled »Moyamoya Disease« by Suzuki and Takaku [287] in the *Archives of Neurology* in 1969, this label has gradually found acceptance throughout the world and is widely used in Japan.

As with the wide variety of names for moyamoya disease, various views concerning its essential nature have been expressed. It has been reported that moyamoya disease is a vascular tumor, since the vascular network is reminiscent of a tumor stain [153, 167, 209, 213]. More frequently, this disease has been considered as a congenital anomaly of the cerebral arteries [2, 65, 99, 119, 150, 184, 213, 210, 257]. A congenital vascular malformation is suggested both by the fact that moyamoya disease has occasionally been found among siblings [213] and by the fact that bilateral lesions are usually found in juvenile cases. From a study of the fetal development of the cerebral vasculature by Padget [239], some researchers have suggested that this disease may be a lesion of the same category as Sturge-Weber disease or Hippel-Lindau disease, based upon the observation that moyamoya vessels resemble those seen at the time of the formation of a plexus-like middle cerebral artery between the anterior branch of the internal carotid artery, including the ophthalmic artery, and the posterior branch, including the posterior communicating artery, when the embryo is between 11 and 12 mm in length. Recently, however, those researchers have tended to favor the collateral pathway hypothesis [206, 304].

From a follow-up angiographical study of young patients, the author [289] has argued that moyamoya disease begins as stenosis of the bilateral terminal portion of the internal carotid artery and gradually progresses to vascular occlusion. In response to this restriction in cerebral blood flow, abnormal net-like vessels are formed at the base of the brain as the collateral pathways. Moreover, dynamic changes in these vessels take place over time. While the causal factors are not known, it is now thought by the majority of researchers that there is an acquired [280, 282], chronic, progressive stenosis of the bilateral terminal portion of the internal carotid artery, although some lateral differences have also been found.

Support for the collateral pathway hypothesis comes from a variety of studies by our group which are discussed in detail in later chapters. These include morphological studies of the perforating arteries in subjects with ages ranging from the fetal stage to adulthood [129, 130], many follow-up studies using cerebral angiography [43, 68, 95, 97, 125, 136, 219, 283, 285, 286, 290, 291, 293], and a vascular structural study involving other organs in the autopsy cases [100]. It can be said that considerable agreement has been reached on these issues in recent years. Indeed, since Kudo's [150] original hypothesis concerning congenital malformation of the circle of Willis, there have appeared numerous reports supporting the acquired theory [142, 145, 147, 149]. And yet, the rare but statistically unlikely occurrence of moyamoya disease in siblings, in cousins, and in parent-and-child certainly suggests the presence of a congenital factor.

It must be considered, however, that if (a) the development of the A_1 portion of the anterior cerebral artery were extremely poor on one side, (b) the other side were normal, and (c) stenosis were to progress due to arteriosclerosis clearly caused by the terminal portion of the internal carotid artery of the good side, then the vascular net at the base of the brain would develop only on the good side. Consequently, unilateral moyamoya vessels must be excluded from consideration of true moyamoya disease. In the case of unilateral abnormalities, it is best to consider such vessels merely as a »moyamoya phenomenon« [309, 312, 315].

Among the causes of moyamoya phenomena which have been reported are the following: von Recklinghausen's disease [336], meningitis tuberculosa, gradual stenosis of the bifurcation of the bilateral terminal portion of the internal carotid artery caused by an enlarging tumor of the pituitary region, and periarteritis nodosa.

Since in adult cases it is thought that moyamoya vessels are occasionally seen due to progressive stenosis caused by arteriosclerosis of the bilateral, intracranial internal carotid arteries, it is essential to differentiate between true moyamoya disease and this type of acquired moyamoya vessels in adults.

In practice, however, it is difficult to distinguish between these two types of lesion, and it is likely that most discussions of moyamoya disease in the literature have been based upon findings both of true moyamoya disease and of moyamoya vessels due to arteriosclerosis. Consequently, when discussing moyamoya disease, it is necessary to exclude moyamoya-like vessels which are thought to be due to clearly anomalous changes in cerebral vessels, such as in the case of arteriovenous malformations.

2 Epidemiology and Symptomatology

2.1 Introduction

Study on the epidemiology of moyamoya disease began in 1965 with a paper concerning 96 cases by Nishimoto et al. [205]. They have since published three additional papers reporting on a total of 518 cases [181]. Various other epidemiological studies have also been undertaken in Japan, notable among these being that of Kudo in 1967 concerning 146 cases [230] and that of Kudo et al. in 1971 concerning 363 cases, all of whom were under the age of 50 years [151]. The research organs of the Japanese Ministry of Health and Welfare also conducted national surveys in 1974–1975 and in 1977–1979. During 1974–1975, some 189 cases of moyamoya disease were found [216] and in 1977–1979 some 590 cases were recorded, a summary of which was published by Yamaguchi et al. [346]. Moreover, Nishimoto et al. have reported a clinical investigation of 389 cases from the 590 reported by Yamaguchi et al. in which all cases of unilateral moyamoya disease and cases in which the condition of the vessels contralateral to moyamoya disease was unknown, were excluded [208].

As is apparent from these reports on moyamoya disease, the total number of moyamoya cases which have been studied is quite large, but the statistical conclusions which have been drawn have been based upon collected data from a wide variety of institutions. Since there remain considerable problems concerning the consistency of diagnosis and differences in the methods of recording anamneses, inevitably the available statistics reveal only the most general trends.

In contrast to the above-mentioned large-scale studies, we have made a detailed investigation of 100 cases experienced in our clinic, where strictly observed criteria for diagnosis and recording of anamneses were used between 1968 and 1980 [93]. Since we believe that the statistical conclusions obtained in that study are more reliable than the statistics from a variety of sources, in the present chapter discussion of the epidemiology of moyamoya disease will be based upon it, with occasional reference to the results obtained in other studies.

2.2 Incidence

The incidence of moyamoya disease is apparently higher in Japan than elsewhere in the world. The relatively high incidence in Japan has frequently been reported since Kudo's early studies [148, 151].

It is important to note that the incidence of moyamoya disease is similar from Hokkaido to Okinawa and that there are no localities within Japan which have unusually high or low incidences. Yamaguchi et al. [346] drew similar conclusions from their study of 519 cases, in which they found a mean incidence of 0.1 cases/100000 people per year in Japan.

Statistical studies of moyamoya disease outside Japan are limited to the one report of Picard et al. [244]. The incidence is apparently lower than that in Japan, but some cases have now been reported in China, Korea, and various countries of Southeast Asia [159], as well as in the United States [248, 339, 342] and Europe [242, 243, 245, 246]. It is worth emphasizing, however, that meaningful discussion of the incidence in countries outside Japan requires that differences in the incidence with which cerebral angiograms are taken also be taken into consideration.

2.3 **Incidence by Sex** (Table 1)

It has been known for some time that moyamoya disease is found more frequently in women than in men [146]. Among our cases as well, a ratio of 1:1.5 (men to women) has been experienced (40 males, 60 females). Study of the incidence by age, however, reveals a different picture. That is, of our 100 cases, 46 were under 15 years of age, while 54 were adult cases (a ratio of 1:1.17). Among juvenile cases only 13 were male, whereas an extremely large number, 33, were female (a ratio of 1:2.53). Among adults, exactly one-half were male and one-half female (27 in each group).

These figures clearly indicate that there is a marked prevalence of moyamoya disease among young females relative to young males, but no such trend is apparent among adult cases.

A tendency for moyamoya disease to occur more frequently in females has been reported by others [148, 151, 346]. The overall ratio of male to female cases varies from 1:1.34 to 1:1.48, whereas among young cases reported ratios range from 1:1.28 to 1:1.59. Among adult cases the mean ratio is said to be 1:1.40.

Table 1. Age and sex distribution. Moyamoya disease is found more frequently in females than in males in all statistics

	Tohoku Univ. (1981)				Kudo (1971)				Nishimoto (1974)				Yamaguchi (1980)			
	M	F	Total	F/M	M	F	Total	F/M	M	F	Total	F/M	M	F	Total	F/M
Juveniles	13	33	46	2.53	63	93	156	1.48	85	135	220	1.59	112	143	255	1.28
Adults	27	27	54	1.0	86	121	207	1.40	124	174	298	1.40	135	189	324	1.40
Unknown													5	6	11	
Total	40	60	100	1.50	149	214	363	1.44	209	309	518	1.48	252	338	590	1.34
Adults/Juveniles	2.07	0.81	1.17		1.37	1.30	1.32		1.46	1.29	1.35		1.21	1.32	1.27	

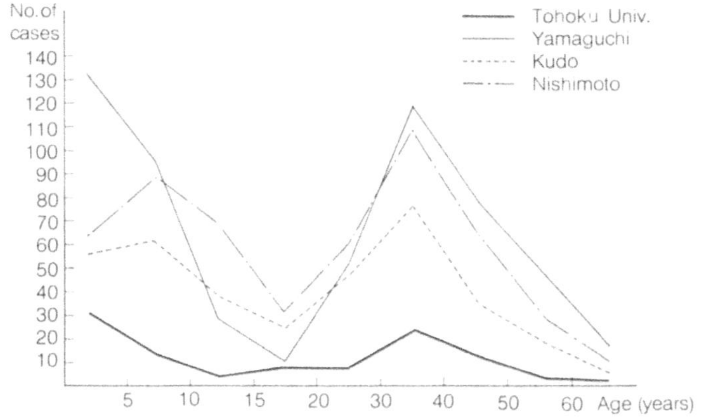

Fig. 2. Age distribution at onset

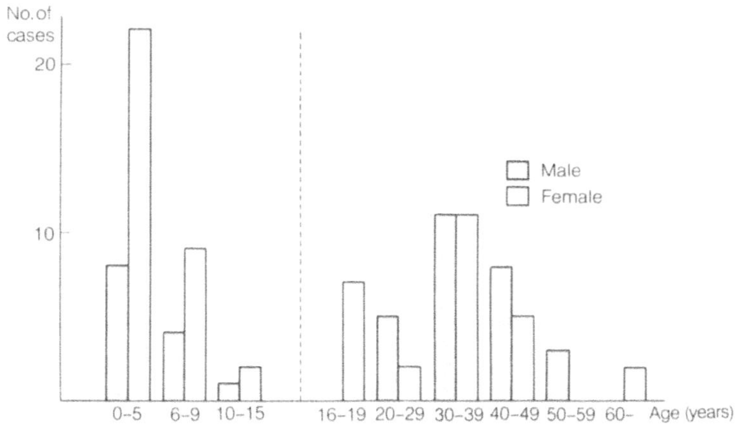

Fig. 3. Age and sex distribution at onset (Tohoku University). Two peaks for the age at onset were observed, between 0 and 5 years and between 30 and 39 years

Empirically, it is evident that moyamoya disease is more frequent in women but the cause for such prevalence remains unclear.

2.4 Age at Onset (Figs. 2, 3)

Study of the age of our patients at the time of onset shows two distinct ages of high prevalence. Among our juvenile cases, 30 were between the ages of 0 and 5 years, 13 were between 6 and 9 years, and 3 were between 10 and 15 years. That is, there was a strong tendency for moyamoya disease to arise in the first 5 years of life – this group accounting for fully 65.2% of our juvenile cases. The average age at onset of juvenile cases was 4.5 years (4.4 years in males and 4.6 years in females).

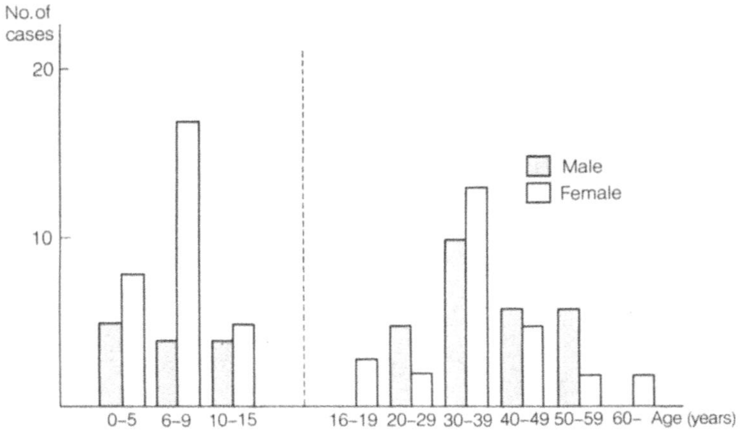

Fig. 4. Age and sex distribution on admission (Tohoku University). The age on admission is approximately the same as the age of onset in adult cases, whereas there is a tendency for admission to be delayed somewhat following onset in juvenile cases

Among adults, there were only seven cases with onset between the ages of 16 and 19 years and seven cases between the ages of 20 and 29 years. In contrast, there were 22 cases between the ages of 30 and 39 years, 13 between 40 and 49 years, 3 between 50 and 59 years, and 2 in patients older than 60 years. Clearly, the 4th decade showed the highest rate of moyamoya disease, the average age being 37.7 years (37.4 in males and 39.0 in females).

To summarize, two peaks for the age at onset have been found — one between 0 and 5 years and the other between 30 and 39 years. Kudo et al. [151] and Nishimoto et al. [205] have reported similar peaks at the ages of 6–10 years and 30–39 years, this being in agreement with our results for adult cases, although they found a somewhat later peak for juvenile cases. It should be noted, however, that Yamaguchi et al. [346] and Nishimoto et al. [218] made further analysis and found two distinct peaks similar to our date — the first at 4–6 years and the second during the 4th decade.

2.5 Age on Admission (Fig. 4)

Few details concerning age on admission have been reported in the literature. In general, the age on admission is approximately the same as the age of onset in adult cases, whereas there is a tendency for admission to be delayed somewhat following onset in juvenile cases.

Among our cases, the age was 0–5 years in 13 cases, 6–9 years in 21 cases, and 10–15 years in 9 cases — showing a peak at the 6- to 9-year period, whereas in adult cases both onset and admission showed peaks late in the 4th decade.

Yamaguchi et al. have reported similar results [346]. The age on admission was 0–4 years in 14.1%, 5–9 years in 17.6%, and 10–14 years in 8.3%; again a peak was apparent at 5–9 years, similar to the results of Nishimoto et al. [208].

The reasons for the slight delay in juvenile cases are thought to include the following. Symptoms in juvenile cases are often transient and many show gradual onset. The child's family is often slow to discover abnormalities, and considerable time is often required to make a definitive diagnosis. In contrast, among adult cases, onset is often accompanied by intracranial hemorrhage, resulting in various acute symptoms, so that onset is followed immediately by admission to hospital.

2.6 Initial Symptoms and Symptoms over the Clinical Course (Fig. 5, Table 2)

Initial symptoms in moyamoya disease (both juvenile and adult cases considered together) are most frequently motor disturbances. Among our cases these were found in 36%, followed by intracranial hemorrhage in 25%, headache in 20%, and convulsions in 6%. These figures are similar to those reported by others. Yamaguchi et al. [346] reported as follows: motor disturbances (62.7% in males, 53.8% in females), disturbances of consciousness (28.1% in males, 34.6% in females), signs of meningeal irritation (10.3% in males, 20.5% in females), and speech disturbances (16.7% in males, 14.0% in females).

When, however, these symptoms are studied with regard to age, large differences between juvenile and adult cases become apparent. Among our juvenile cases, motor disturbances, including monoparesis, paraparesis, and

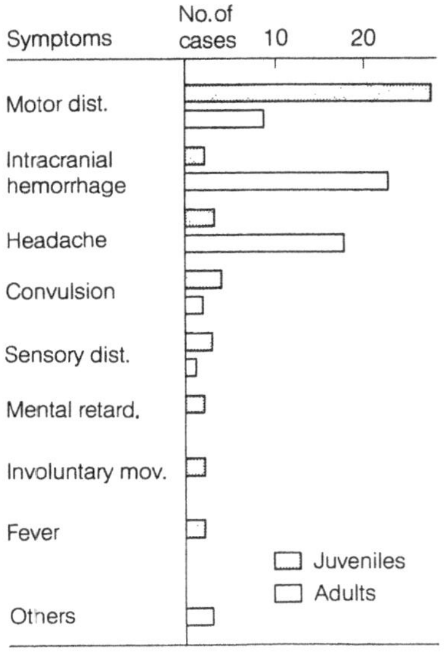

Fig. 5. Initial symptoms (Tohoku University). As initial symptoms, motor disturbances in juvenile cases and intracranial hemorrhages in adult cases were frequently observed

Table 2. Symptoms over the clinical course of juvenile and adult cases. The incidence of these symptoms is very similar to the incidence of those at onset

Symptoms	Juveniles	Adults
Motor disturbance	44	16
Sensory disturbance	8	10
Intracranial hemorrhage	2	23
Headache	8	11
Convulsion	14	3
Speech disturbance	15	8
Involuntay movement	8	2
Visual disturbance	6	6
Mental deficit, psychic disturbance	13	8
Conscious disturbance	3	12
Vertigo	2	2
Dysphagia	1	1
Apraxia	1	1

hemiparesis, were found in 28 of 46 cases (60%). Among those 46 cases, some 20 % showed motor disturbances indicative of transient brain ischemia. If one also includes other symptoms thought to be due to brain ischemia, such as sensory disturbances and mental and psychic disorders (75), then 85% of these cases (39 of 46 juvenile cases) showed symptoms of brain ischemia. These symptoms often are induced by crying, blowing, and so-called hyperventilation [9, 135].

Intracranial hemorrhage was seen in only two juvenile cases (4%), whereas among adult cases onset was accompanied by intracranial hemorrhage in 23 cases (43%) [71, 80]. Symptoms due to brain ischemia [222], including motor, mental, and psychic disturbances [67, 75], were seen in relatively few cases (11 of 54 cases or 20%).

These findings concerning symptomatology are virtually identical to those of other writers. That is, juvenile cases are often said to begin with transient motor disturbances, i.e., symptoms of transient brain ischemia. Paresis is usually ipsilateral, but there are a variety of other types, such as cases in which paresis changes to the contralateral side and cases in which paresis becomes bilateral.

As we have previously reported [133, 296], most adult moyamoya cases show intracranial hemorrhage, but it is not normally subarachnoid hemorrhage from moyamoya vessels at the base of the brain. Rather there are thought to be two main mechanisms of onset: most commonly, ventricular hemorrhage caused by rupture into the lateral ventricles of an intracerebral hematoma located somewhere around these ventricles; and, less commonly, subarachnoid hemorrhage due to rupture of a basilar artery aneurysm.

In general, the symptoms which appear over the duration of the clinical course and their incidence are very similar to those at onset. In juvenile cases, however, it is often found that repeated convulsions eventually lead to mental deterioration [357].

2.7 Laboratory Findings on Admission (Table 3)

We undertake general laboratory tests of all our adult and juvenile cases of moyamoya disease at the time of admission. Although a full test battery is obtained whenever possible, no clear trends in laboratory data have emerged. We now believe that there is a need for detailed immunological and other specialized tests in such patients, but sufficient data are not yet available.

2.8 Family History

Among our 100 cases of moyamoya disease, we have experienced three cases in which the patient had a parent, sibling, or identical twin with the same disease [273, 276, 345]. One other of our patients had a sibling with a history of periarteritis nodosa.

In general, most of the reports of moyamoya disease among family members have been concerned with siblings [123, 201, 272]. Takeuchi [310] reported 4 pairs (8 moyamoya cases) among 118 cases in the literature and Kudo et al. [151] reported 7 pairs (14 cases) among 363 cases in the literature, as well as one uncle–nephew pair. Nishimoto [204] found 7 pairs (14 cases) among 518 cases queried by written questionnaire. Finally, from 590 cases investigated by questionnaire, Yamaguchi et al. [346] found 12 pairs (24 cases) which were thought to be intrafamilial – fully 10 of which were siblings. The remaining two pairs were a mother and child and the relationship between two of the cases remains uncertain.

These findings suggest, however, that the incidence of moyamoya disease among related family members is not particularly high. Various authors have previously emphasized the fact of occasional intrafamilial occurrence and argued

Table 3. Laboratory findings on admission. No abnormal data were observed

Hematological examination
Blood picture
Hemorrhagic diathesis
Blood sedimentation rate
Serological examinations
Serum electrolytes
Serum proteins
Serum lipids
Liver function
Renal function
Rheumatoid arthritis, antistreptolysin-O,
C-reactive protein
Hepatitis B antigen
Wassermann's reaction, etc.
Urinary examinations
Cerebrospinal fluid examinations
Others

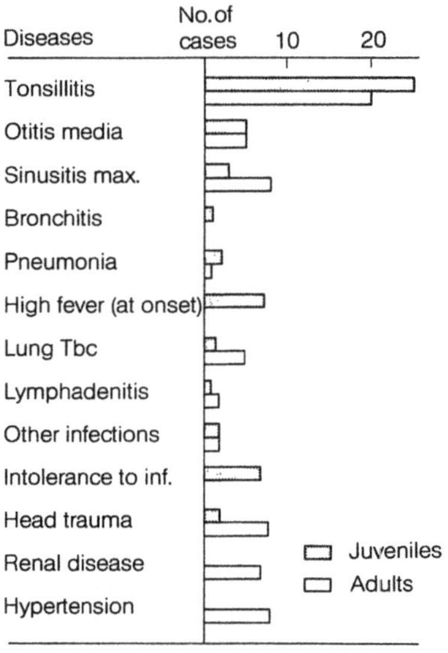

Fig. 6. Past history of moyamoya disease (Tohoku University). A history of tonsillitis was characteristically found in 65% of juvenile cases and 40% of adult cases

that moyamoya disease is a congenital or genetic anomaly, but from the above figures it is apparent that isolated occurrence is far more frequently seen. It is now apparent that more emphasis should be placed on investigation into the predispositional factors which are associated with a tendency toward contraction of moyamoya disease, rather than on strictly genetic factors.

A number of studies have also appeared in the literature reporting moyamoya cases with family members suffering from cerebral aneurysms, cerebral arteriovenous malformation, or subarachnoid hemorrhage of unknown cause, but no notable correlation has been found between moyamoya disease and any other known anomaly.

2.9 **Anamnesis** (Fig. 6)

When studying the nature and causal factors in moyamoya disease, it is important to study carefully the patient's anamnesis. Among our 100 cases, a history of tonsillitis was the most frequently encountered — found in 65% of juvenile cases and 40% of adult cases. Among those with a history of tonsillitis, a history of repeated tonsillitis was not uncommon. Furthermore, among the cases with apparently normal tonsils, a few cases were found to have pus in the posterior part of the tonsils. These findings concerning tonsillitis are somewhat at odds with the anamnesis data in other reports, but the fact that our cases were examined by similar means in the same clinic and that great care was taken in recording the patient's medical history suggests that our data concerning inflammation of the tonsils may be important.

We have also found that a majority of moyamoya patients have had histories of repeated infection above the neck region. Among juvenile cases, 34 (74%) had had sinusitis, otitis media, or other inflammation above the neck including tonsillitis. Among adult cases, 26 (46%) had had similar infections of the head. Furthermore, seven of the juvenile cases were notable in the fact that they easily succumbed to common infectious diseases. Finally, among the adult cases, seven had renal disease and eight (including four with renal disease) had hypertension.

In a study concerning cases from various clinics, Kudo et al. [151] reported that moyamoya patients included a small number with nephritis, tonsillitis, or tuberculosis, and there have also been cases of some patients who have shown the onset of moyamoya disease having had a fever previously and following a fever having developed in reaction to prophylactic injections. He did not, however, discuss the incidence of such cases.

In an investigation of 85 cases with well-documented histories, Yamaguchi et al. [346] found 32 with inflammation of the upper respiratory tract. Bacterial infections, such as tonsillitis (4 cases), inflammation of the face and the neck (5 cases), appendicitis, otitis media, and sinusitis were found in 22 cases. In other words, a total of 54 cases (63.5%) showed infections of some kind and a majority of these were infections above the neck. Such findings are thought to suggest the involvement of inflammatory disease above the neck in the genesis of moyamoya disease [137, 281].

Head trauma was found in eight of our cases (8%) and in eight of Yamaguchi's cases (9.4%), but the causal relationship between trauma and moyamoya disease is uncertain. The presence of other diseases or congenital anomalies has been reported in the literature [42, 90, 103, 200, 279], but again causal relations remain unknown.

2.10 Conclusion

We have discussed the epidemiology of moyamoya disease both in the light of our own experiences with 100 cases and those reported in the literature. Since our 100 cases have all been experienced in the same clinic using consistent diagnostic methods, the results obtained are thought to have statistical significance superior to the conclusions drawn from data obtained from a multitude of disparate sources.

Moyamoya disease is found throughout Japan without any locations of unusual incidence. An incidence of 0.1 cases/100000 people per year has been reported.

This vascular anomaly is more frequently found in females, and there are two periods of relatively high incidence – between the ages of 0 and 5 years and during the 4th decade. The age on admission is virtually the same as that at onset in adult cases, whereas there is a slight delay between onset and hospitalization in juvenile cases. Among juvenile cases, the symptoms seen at onset and throughout the clinical course are generally those due to transient brain ischemia, whereas among adult cases symptoms are generally those due to intracranial hemorrhage. There is, in fact, general agreement in the literature concerning the symptomatology of this disease.

It is particularly noteworthy that among our 100 cases of moyamoya disease, a history of infections above the neck, especially tonsillitis, was often found.

3 Cerebral Angiography

3.1 Introduction

Patients with moyamoya disease display characteristic clinical symptoms and, as discussed in Chap. 5, characteristic EEG records are also found. Definitive diagnosis, however, is possible only by means of cerebral angiography. Cerebral angiograms in moyamoya disease show various features [41, 62, 125, 136, 287, 289, 293] which are, interestingly, different in juvenile and adult cases. In juvenile cases, sequential angiograms show dynamic changes with time, but in the early stages of the disease such small changes are often overlooked. It is therefore important to understand thoroughly angiographical findings at all stages in the course of moyamoya disease.

In this chapter, the characteristic findings of angiograms in moyamoya disease, including basal moyamoya [287, 289], ethmoidal moyamoya [283, 293], and vault moyamoya [136] are discussed with particular emphasis on the differences between juvenile and adult moyamoya disease and the reason for the differences.

3.2 Basal Moyamoya

3.2.1 Angiographical Follow-up of Juvenile Cases and a Six-Stage Classification of the Process of Change

Suzuki et al. [289] reported details of carotid angiograms obtained in a follow-up study of four of their ten juvenile cases of moyamoya disease in which bilateral cerebral angiograms were taken. The initial change is stenosis of the terminal bifurcation of the bilateral internal carotid artery (ICA). Thereafter, the stenosis gradually progresses and an abnormal network of vessels at the base of the brain (basal moyamoya) appears (Fig. 7). Sequential changes are then found in these abnormal vessels, as reported by Suzuki et al. in 1965 [289]. In that report, a six-stage classification of moyamoya disease was introduced based upon the sequential changes in cerebral angiograms of basal moyamoya.

The six stages were as follows:

Stage 1. Narrowing of the carotid fork (Fig. 8). This is a stage during which there is only mild stenosis of the carotid fork, with no other angiographical changes apparent.

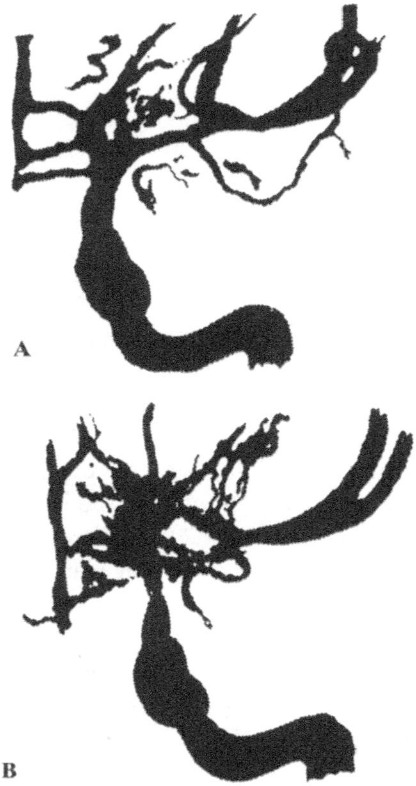

Fig. 7. A Left carotid angiogram, anteroposterior view, just after onset. Slight stenotic change is observed around the carotid fork. **B** Carotid angiogram of the same patient taken 9 months after onset. Stenosis at the carotid fork had progressed and basal moyamoya had appeared

Stage 2. Initiation of moyamoya (dilatation of all the main cerebral arteries) Fig. 9). During this stage, the carotid fork is not so narrow; rather all the main cerebral arteries dilate, and very slight moyamoya vessels appear only near the carotid fork itself.

Stage 3. Intensification of moyamoya [disappearance of the middle cerebral artery (MCA) and the anterior cerebral artery (ACA)] (Fig. 10).

By this stage, distinct moyamoya vessels are apparent at the base of the brain. Such moyamoya vessels are individually quite thick and distinct. Moreover, defects in the main intracerebral arteries, such as the MCA and ACA, begin to be visible and vessels appear which are thought to be collateral pathways from the external carotid arterial system to the brain.

Stage 4. Minimization of moyamoya [disappearance of the posterior cerebral artery (PCA)] (Fig. 11).

Should the posterior communicating arteries be congenitally small or defective, naturally the PCA would not be visualized from the beginning. In this

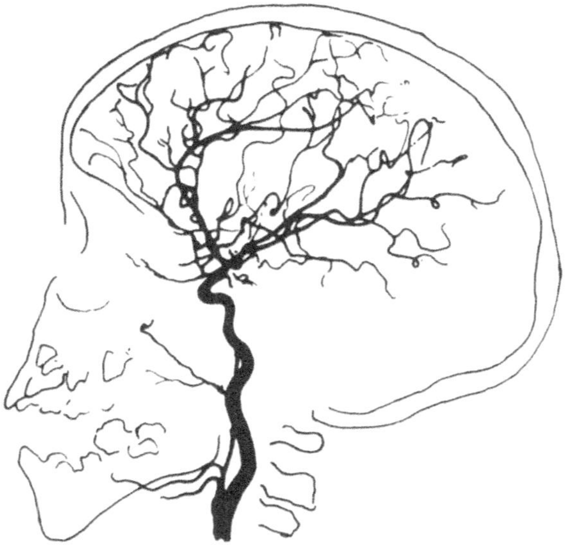

Fig. 8. Stage 1: Narrowing of the carotid fork. Only the carotid fork stenosis is observed

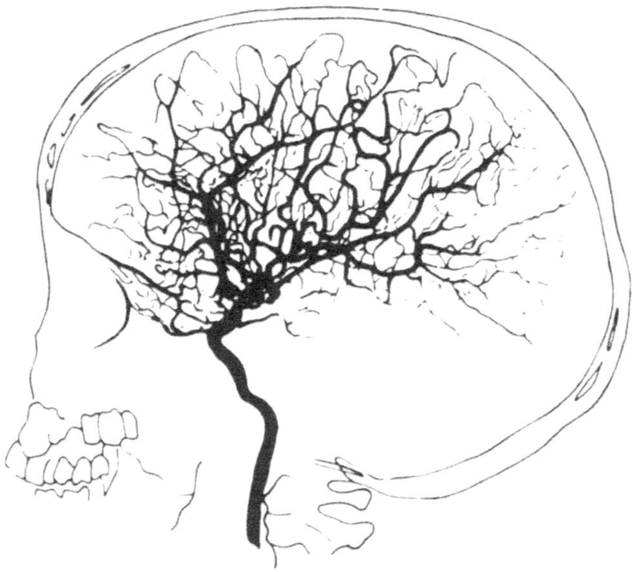

Fig. 9. Stage 2: Initiation of moyamoya. The carotid fork stenosis and very slight basal moyamoya are found. Dilatation of all the main cerebral arteries is also observed

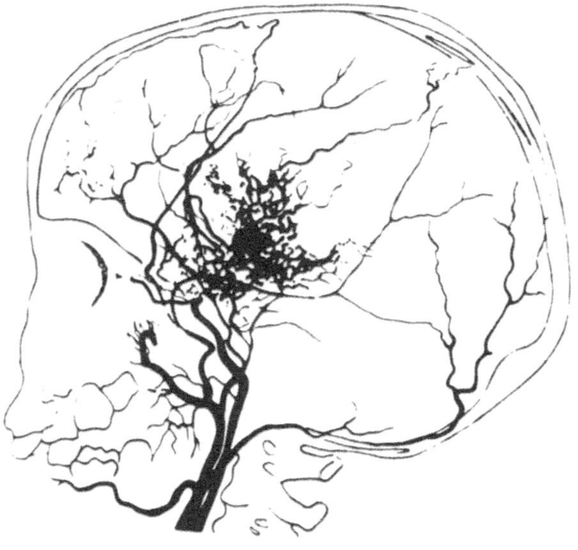

Fig. 10. Stage 3: Intensification of moyamoya. Remarkable moyamoya vessels at the base of the brain. Such moyamoya vessels are individually quite thick and distinct. Moreover, the disappearance of the middle and anterior cerebral arteries begin to be observed

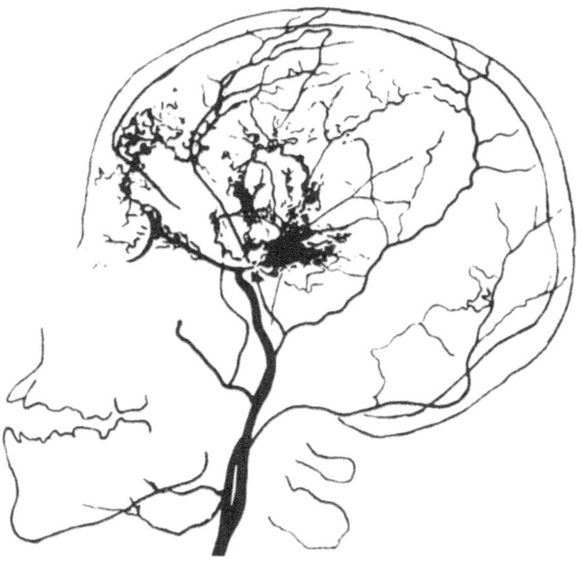

Fig. 11. Stage 4: Minimization of moyamoya. The moyamoya vessels become narrow and form a poor network at the base of the brain. Neither the anterior nor the middle cerebral artery are visualized. Moyamoya vessels at the ethmoidal sinus (ethmoidal moyamoya) conversely increase

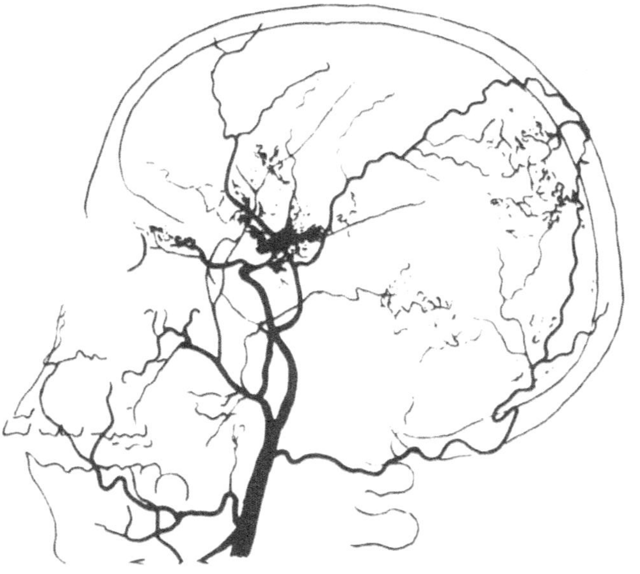

Fig. 12. Stage 5: Reduction of moyamoya. Moyamoya vessels at the base of the brain will be further narrowed and localized to the vicinity of the carotid siphon. There is also an increase in the collateral pathways from the external carotid arterial system

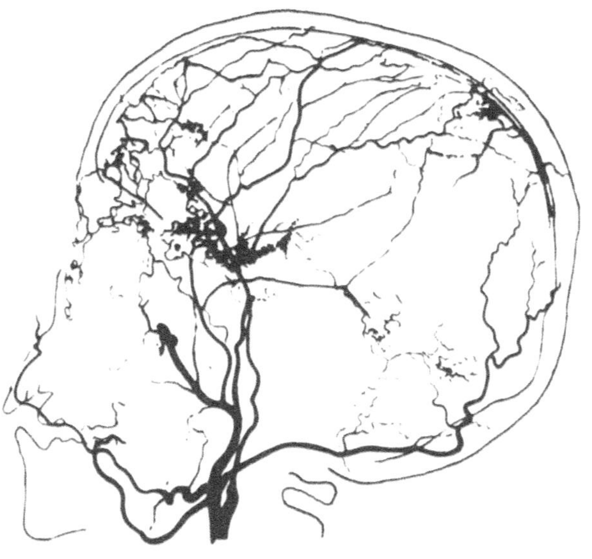

Fig. 13. Stage 6: Disappearance of moyamoya. All of the main arteries arising from the internal carotid arterial system and moyamoya vessels completely disappear in angiograms. The cerebrum is maintained only by means of blood flowing from the external carotid or the vertebral arterial system

stage, occlusion of the ICA extends as far as the junction of the posterior communicating artery, and finally the PCA which has been visualized so far will disappear from the angiogram.

However, even during this period, the ACA and MCA can be traced very dimly or in a completely different shape through the mist of the moyamoya vessels. Moreover, the moyamoya vessels become coarse during this stage, constituent vessels becoming narrow and forming a poor network at the base of the brain. Ethmoidal moyamoya, described below, conversely increases, and the collaterals from the extracranial vessels also enlarge gradually.

Stage 5. Reduction of moyamoya (disappearance of all the main cerebral arteries) (Fig. 12). During this stage, all of the main arteries arising from the internal carotid arterial system nearly disappear in angiograms, there is further minimization of moyamoya vessels, and the moyamoya vessels are found localized to the vicinity of the carotid siphon. The obstruction further extends downward, showing a complete occlusion as far as C_2 or to below C_3 in the ICA. There is also an increase in the collateral pathways from the external carotid arterial system.

Stage 6. Disappearance of moyamoya (cerebral blood is supplied only from the external carotid artery and the vertebral arteries) (Fig. 13).

There is complete disappearance of the ICA siphon region in angiograms and nearly complete disappearance of the moyamoya vessels at the base of the brain. Only collateral pathways from the external carotid arterial system are seen to enter the brain. Cerebral blood flow from the internal carotid arterial system is completely halted and the cerebrum is maintained only by means of blood flowing from the external carotid system and the vertebral arterial system.

3.2.2 Long-term Follow-up of Juvenile Cases

We have performed sequential follow-up studies of bilateral carotid angiograms in nine juvenile cases, extending over several years. The shortest period for such a follow-up was 5 years and 11 months, whereas the longest period was 18 years and 3 months. In 17 of the 18 sides from the 9 cases, the above-described process of moyamoya development was observed (Fig. 14). In previous reports, even where follow-up studies were carried out, few changes with time have been noted. Our studies, in contrast, have shown that, while there are also cases of dynamic changes over a short time interval, it is unlikely that the progressive development of moyamoya disease through all six stages will be found unless long-term follow-up is undertaken. This is inevitable, since many cases proceed by only one stage over a period of up to 10 years.

Here a typical case which we were able to follow for 18 years is presented. This male patient was studied from the time when his initial right carotid angiograms showed almost no vascular abnormality until the full development of the disease bilaterally.

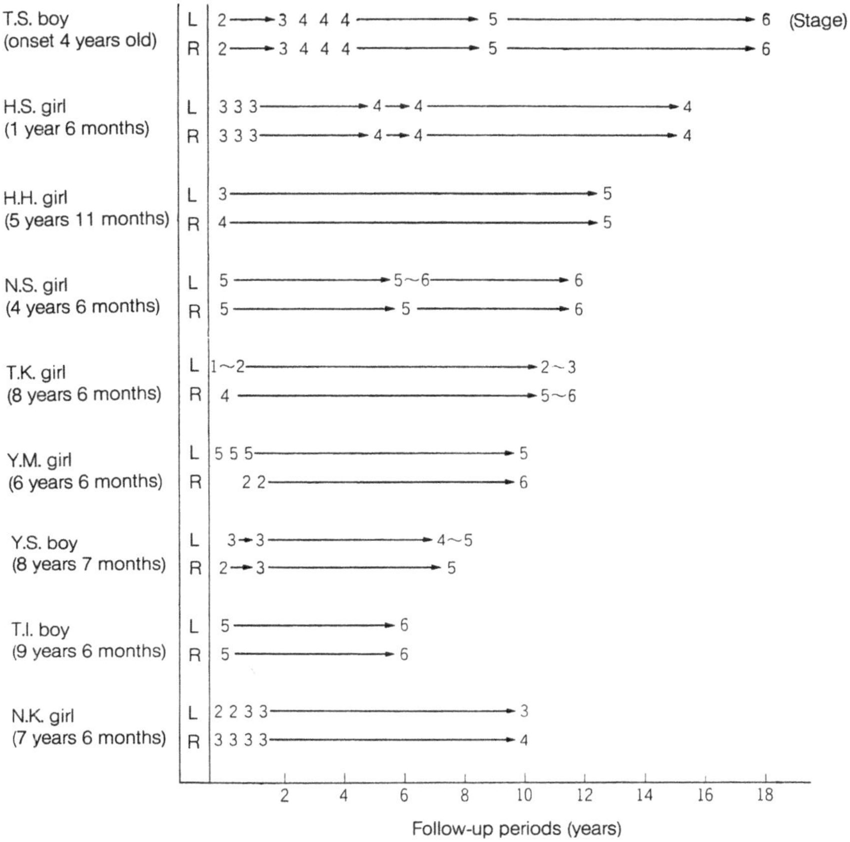

Fig. 14. Sequential follow-up studies on changes of the cerebral arteries by bilateral carotid angiograms in juvenile cases. The shortest follow-up period was 5 years and 11 months, whereas the longest period was 18 years and 3 months. In 17 out of the 18 examined sides from the 9 cases, their stages had progressed

He was first examined at the age of 4 years and was followed until the age of 22 years. Sudden right-sided hemiparesis and speech disturbances were noted on 25 January 1964. He was examined in hospital, but all symptoms disappeared shortly thereafter (within 5 h). The initial right carotid angiograms (Fig. 15), obtained on 31 January 1964, showed slight stenosis of the terminal portion of the ICA, possibly slight dilatation of the trunk arteries of the brain, and a suggestion of fine moyamoya vessels at the base of the brain, but these findings were nearly normal in most respects (stage 2).

A second right carotid angiogram was obtained on 12 October 1965, 1 year and 9 months subsequent to the initial angiography (Fig. 16). The lateral view showed large differences from the earlier angiograms. At the base of the brain there were marked moyamoya vessels and the MCA had already disappeared from the

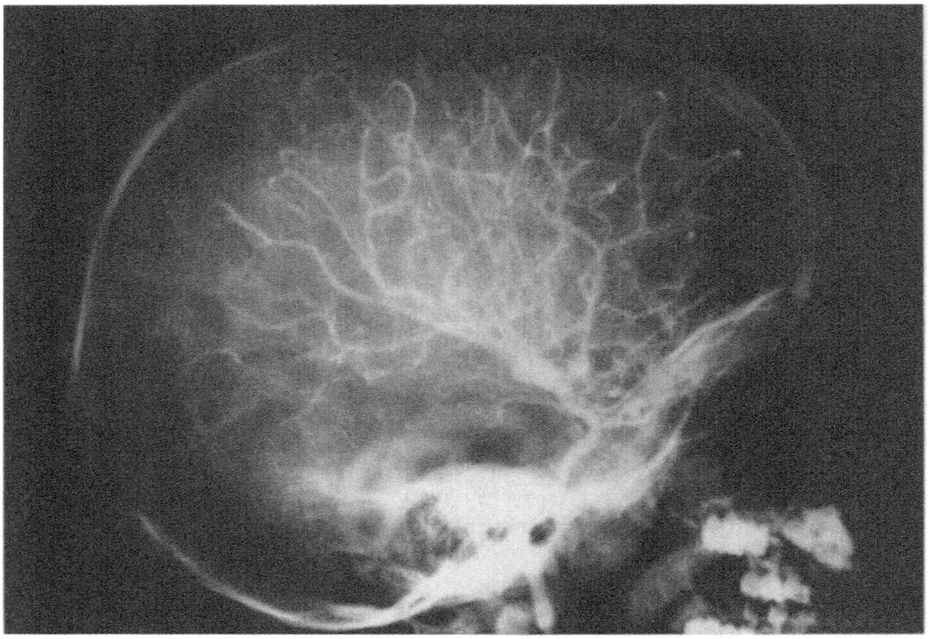

Fig. 15. First right carotid angiogram, lateral view, of a 4-year-old boy. Slight stenosis at the carotid fork without basal moyamoya and dilated cerebral arteries were revealed (stage 2)

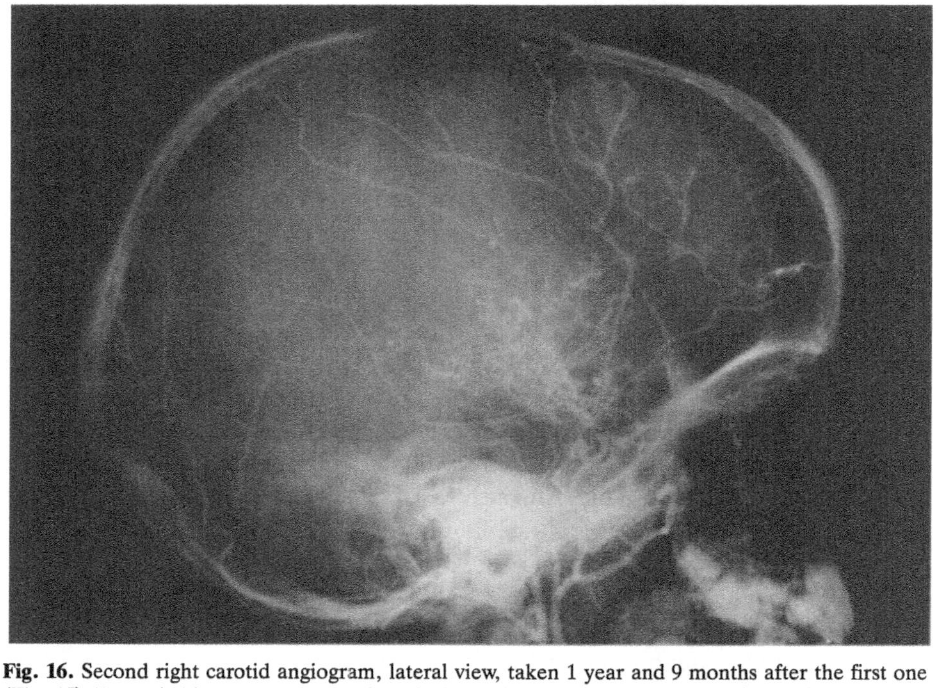

Fig. 16. Second right carotid angiogram, lateral view, taken 1 year and 9 months after the first one (Fig. 15). Remarkable moyamoya vessels at the base of the brain were observed (stage 3)

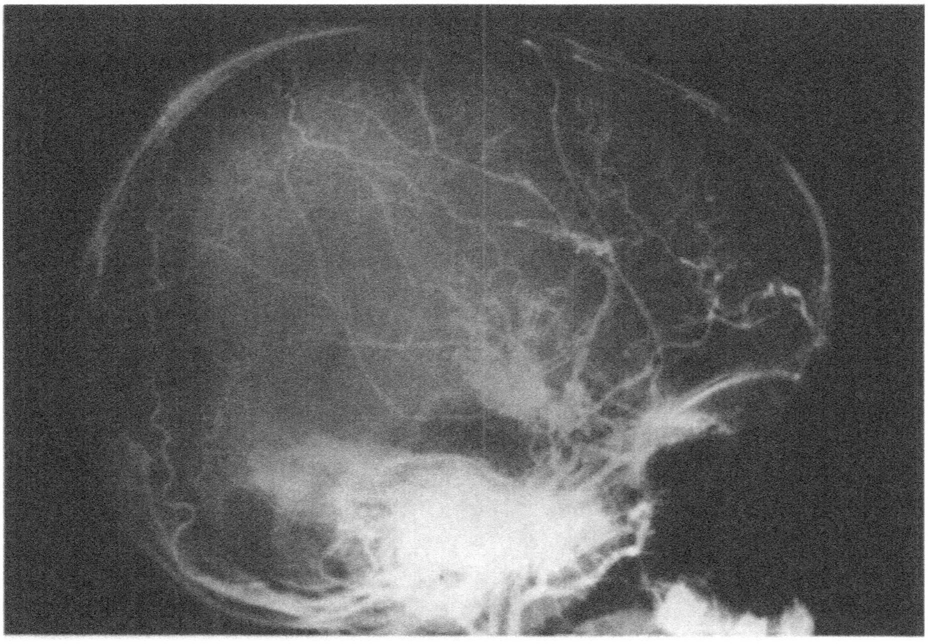

Fig. 17. Third right carotid angiogram taken 2 years and 7 months after the first one (Fig. 15). The basal moyamoya vessels were seen to be reduced (stage 4)

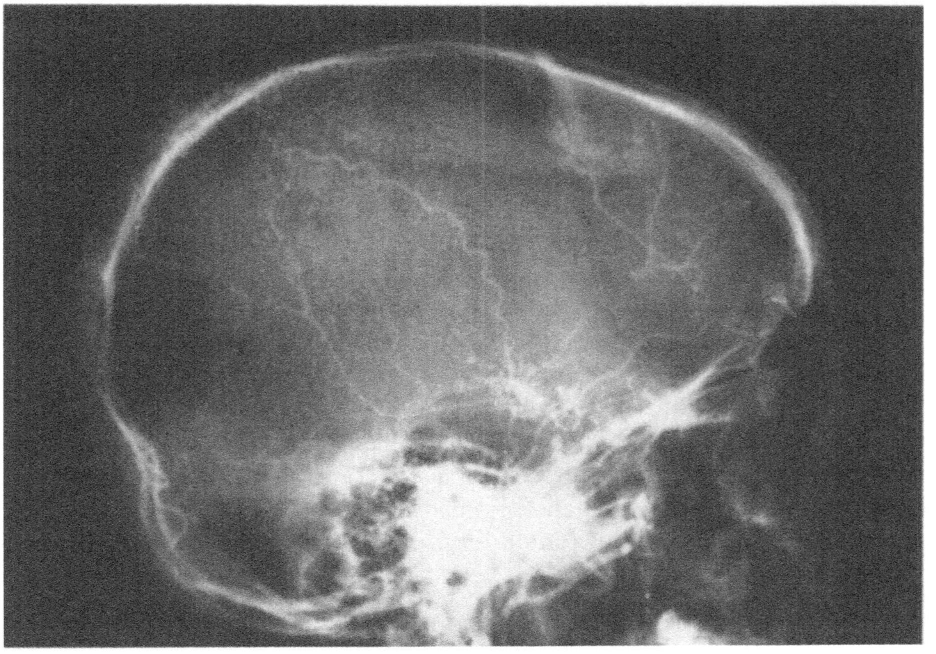

Fig. 18. Fourth right carotid angiogram taken 9 years and 2 months after the first one (Fig. 15). Reduction of basal moyamoya vessels and defection of the whole main cerebral arteries were seen. The external carotid arterial system became dominant (stage 5)

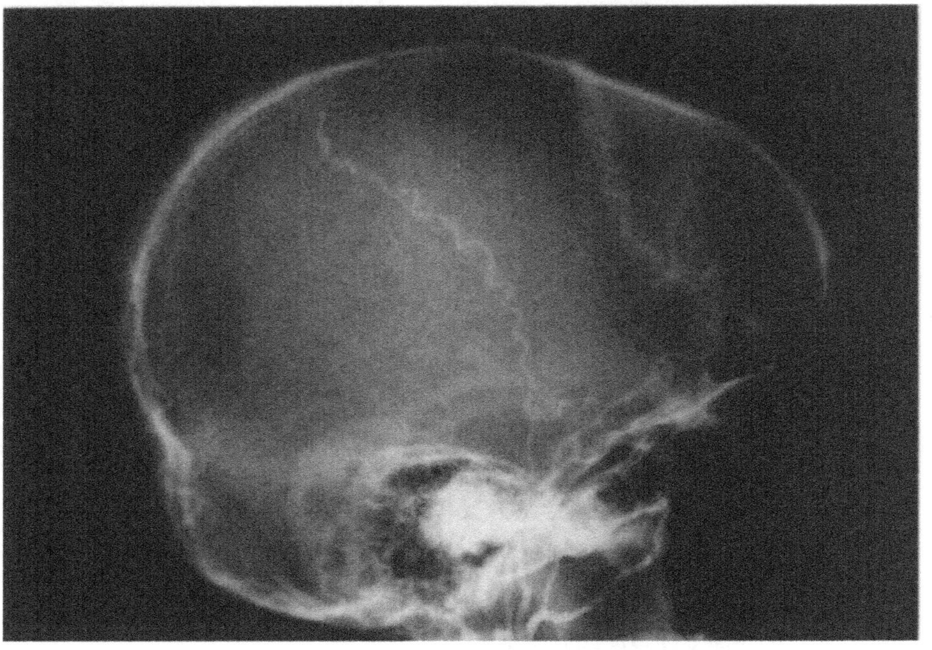

Fig. 19. Fifth right carotid angiogram taken 18 years and 3 months after the first one (Fig. 15). Almost all basal moyamoya disappeared and blood was supplied to branches of the anterior cerebral artery via the external carotid arterial system (stage 6)

angiogram (Fig. 16), although the ACA remained. In an anterior-posterior view, however, the MCA was found to remain and, although narrow, it was visible as far as its peripheral portions (stage 3).

Right carotid angiograms were obtained again on 1 August 1966, 2 years and 7 months after first examination (Fig. 17). In a lateral view, the basal moyamoya vessels were seen to be reduced and the MCA was visible, if only barely (stage 4).

Angiography was performed again on 31 March 1973, 9 years and 2 months following the first examination (Fig. 18). The ICA had become narrow rostral from the cervical bifurcation. Occlusion was seen in the carotid fork region, above which there was slight basal moyamoya (stage 5).

Right carotid angiograms were again obtained on 21 April 1982, 18 years and 3 months subsequent to the first examination (Fig. 19). Almost all the basal moyamoya had disappeared and moyamoya vessels of the cranial vault region, passing from the external carotid artery (i. e., vault moyamoya) could be seen (stage 6).

3.2.3 Follow-up of Adult Cases

In marked contrast to juvenile cases, where clear changes in the vasculature of the brain in moyamoya disease can often be seen, there is virtually no change seen in the angiograms of adult patients (Figs. 20, 21). This fact strongly suggests that moyamoya disease in adults is fundamentally different from moyamoya disease in children and that the causal factors are also somehow different. It is also thought that among adult cases are some cases in which the onset of symptoms occurred during adulthood, although the moyamoya disease itself had developed from childhood, progressed to a certain stage, and then remained at that stage until adulthood.

3.3 Nature of Basal Moyamoya

As mentioned above, various views concerning the nature of basal moyamoya have been expressed. The author has maintained that moyamoya vessels are produced in response to chronic, progressive stenotic changes in the intracranial ICA and that they are collateral pathways from the perforating arteries at the base of the brain [280, 285, 286, 287, 288, 289, 290]. There have been few reports concerning whether or not the perforating arteries could give rise to collateral pathways and, therefore, many uncertainties remain [24, 104, 105, 118, 232, 265]. Furthermore, although there are clear quantitative and qualitative differences in the nature and sequential changes of the moyamoya vessels in children and adults, it is uncertain whether or not there are anatomical grounds which could explain those differences.

In order to resolve some of these questions, Kodama [129, 130] made a microangiographical study and undertook the reconstruction of cerebral blood vessels using fetal, juvenile, and adult autopsy material. Specifically, investigation was made of the changes with aging of the middle striate artery, which is the largest branch among the basal perforating branches. A study was also made of the presence of anastomosis between peripheral branches and their changes with aging — that is, the possibility of collateral pathways from the perforating arteries at the base of the brain.

3.3.1 Changes with Aging in the Middle Striate Artery

In light of the fact that there are gradual morphological changes in the middle striate arteries (MSA) with aging (Fig. 22), especially a reduction in the number of such arteries (Fig. 23), it was considered that advancing age may reduce the need for blood vessels which are required during the fetal and childhood stages when brain growth is rapid. This, in effect, would produce a state of functional obstruction. If this phenomenon is then considered in terms of collateral pathways, formation of collateral pathways during obstruction of trunk arteries of the brain, as in moyamoya disease, should be easier in young individuals when the number of vessels is greater and, moreover, the capacity for forming collateral vessels should decrease with age.

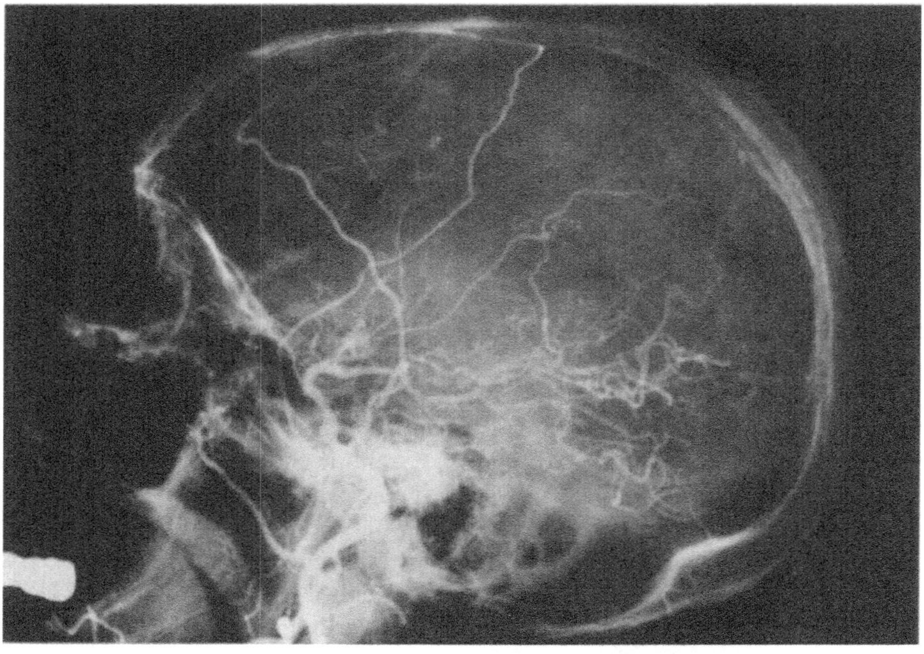

Fig. 20. Left carotid angiogram of a 54-year-old male patient taken just after onset

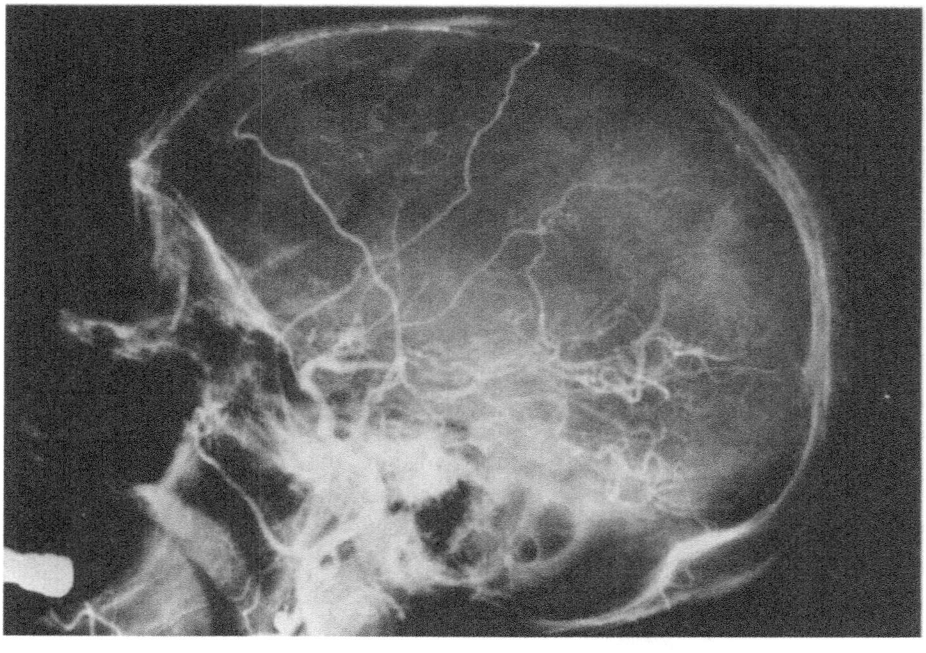

Fig. 21. Left carotid angiogram of the same patient as in Fig. 20 taken 2 years after onset. Changes of basal moyamoya were hardly seen

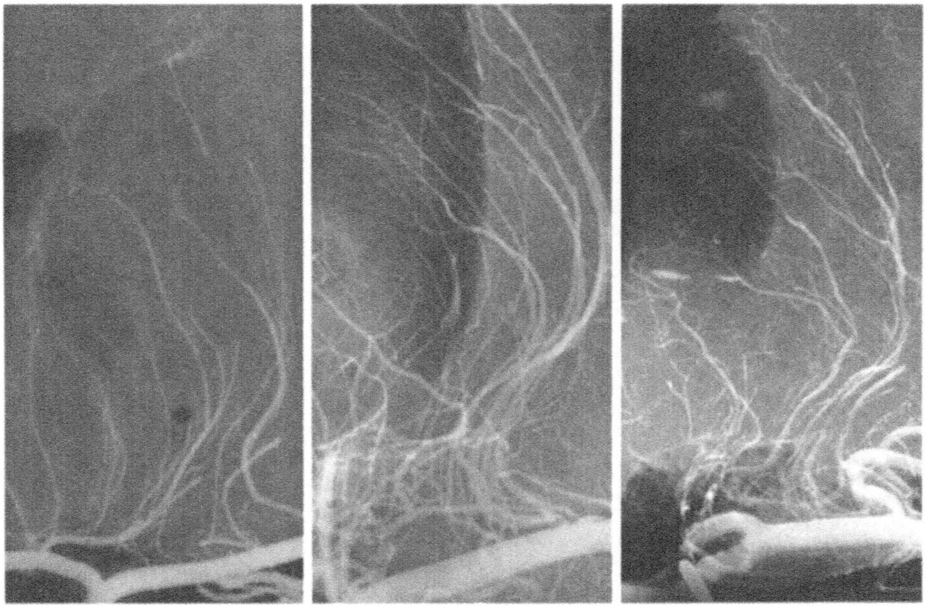

A, B C

Fig. 22 A–C. Changes of course and shape in the middle striate arteries with aging. **A** Normal brain of a fetus (6 months); **B** normal brain of a child (6 years); **C** normal brain of an adult (60 years)

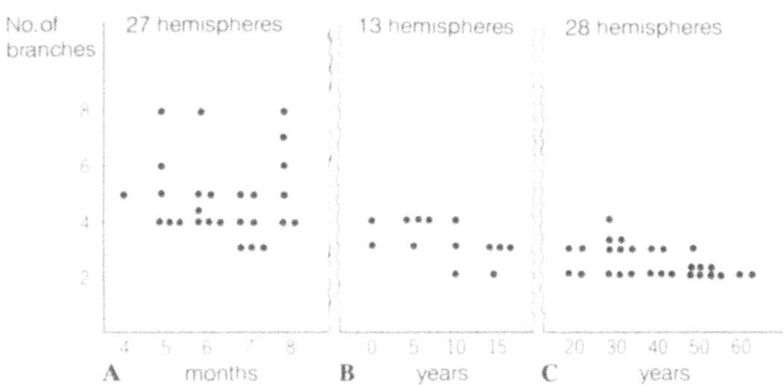

Fig. 23 A–C. Changes in the number of the middle striate arteries with aging. **A** Normal fetus (average = 4.9); **B** normal children (average = 3.2); **C** normal adults (average = 2.4)

3.3.2 Anastomosis Among Peripheral Branches of the Middle Striate Arteries

Based on the fact that, at the capillary level, there clearly is anastomosis between branches of the MSA [129, 130, 300] (Figs. 24–26) and between the MSA and medullary arteries [100, 129, 130, 220, 300] (Figs. 27–31), we believe that such anastomotic branches may function as collateral pathways and that the diameter of these branches is larger and the formation of collateral pathways easier, the younger the individual.

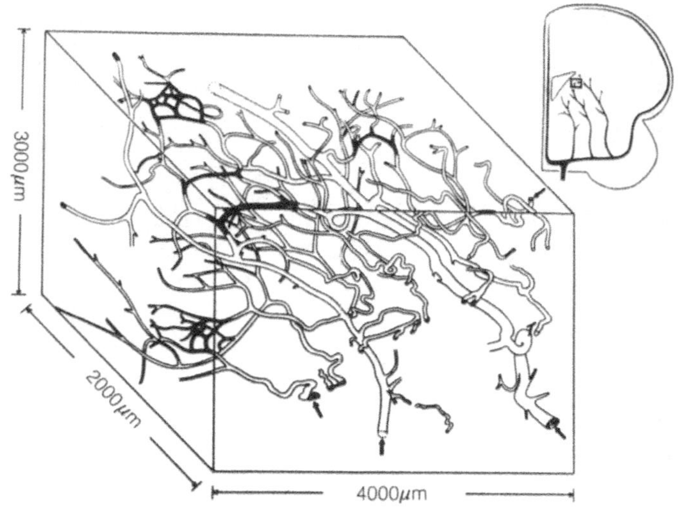

Fig. 24. Normal fetus (5 months). Anastomoses among peripheral branches of the middle striate arteries. The anastomosing pattern is reticular type and H-shaped (*black line*). Maximum diameter of anastomosing branch is 50 μm

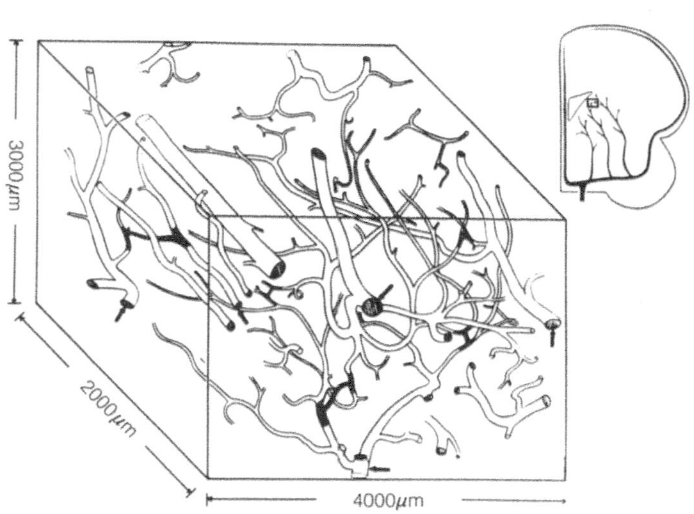

Fig. 25. Normal child (6 years). Anastomoses among peripheral branches of the middle striate arteries. The anastomosing pattern is H-shaped (*black line*). Maximum diameter of anastomosing branch is 30 μm

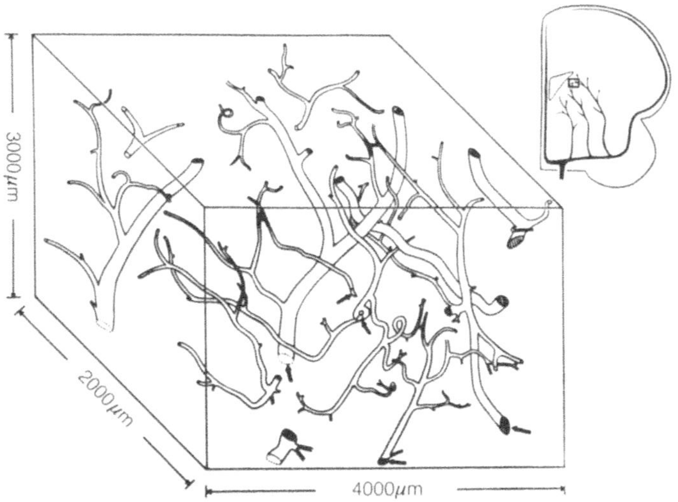

Fig. 26. Normal adult (32 years). Anastomoses among peripheral branches of the middle striate arteries. The anastomosing pattern is H-shaped (*black line*) and the vascular density becomes less than that of a child. Maximum diameter of the anastomosing branch is 20 μm

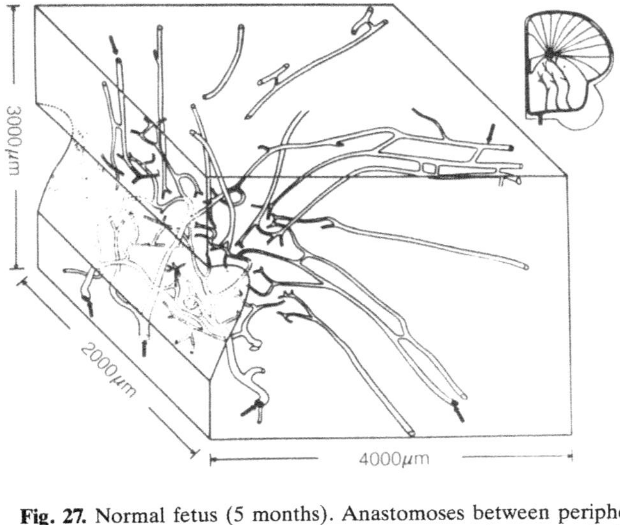

Fig. 27. Normal fetus (5 months). Anastomoses between peripheral branches of the middle striate arteries and the medullary arteries. The anastomosing pattern is divided into two groups; end-to-end and end-to-side anastomoses (*black line*). There was no reticular type of anastomoses such as that seen in perforating arteries. Maximum diameter of anastomosing branch is about 35 μm

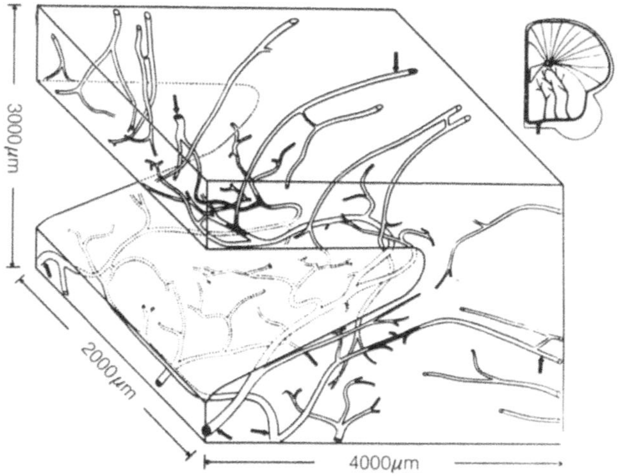

Fig. 28. Normal child (6 years). Anastomoses between peripheral branches of the middle striate arteries and the medullary arteries. The anastomosing pattern is similar to that of a fetus and maximum diameter of anastomosing branch is 30 μm

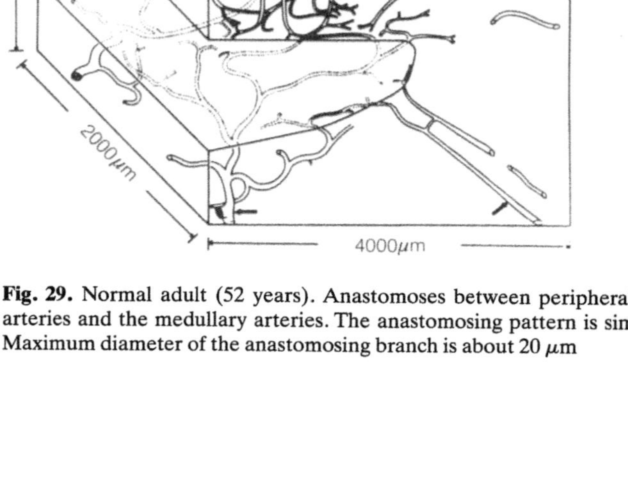

Fig. 29. Normal adult (52 years). Anastomoses between peripheral branches of the middle striate arteries and the medullary arteries. The anastomosing pattern is similar to that of a fetus and child. Maximum diameter of the anastomosing branch is about 20 μm

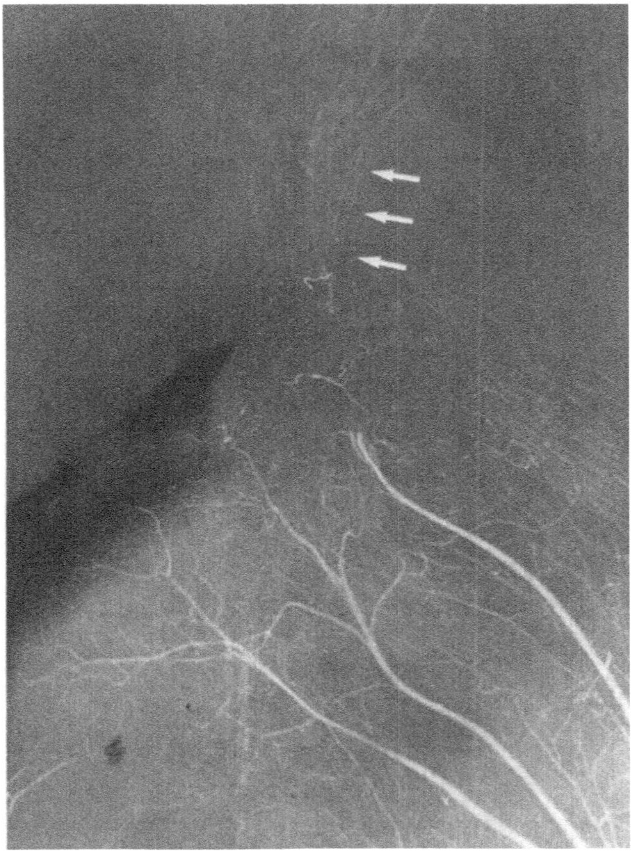

Fig. 30. Normal fetus (7 months). Flow of contrast media from the perforating branches of the middle cerebral artery to the medullary arteries (*arrows*)

These morphological considerations alone may explain the differences in the nature of moyamoya vessels in juvenile and adult cases. Moreover, this view of moyamoya disease strongly suggests that the lesion is a type of collateral pathway arising primarily from the perforating arteries.

3.4 Ethmoidal Moyamoya

In lateral views of carotid angiograms in cases of moyamoya disease, basal moyamoya-like vessels can be seen at the roof of the orbit. These vessels are not composed of the intraorbital vessels, but of dilated vessels on the mucous membrane of the ethmoidal sinus and upper nasal meatus. Thus, this state will hence be called ethmoidal moyamoya (Figs. 32, 33) [283, 293].

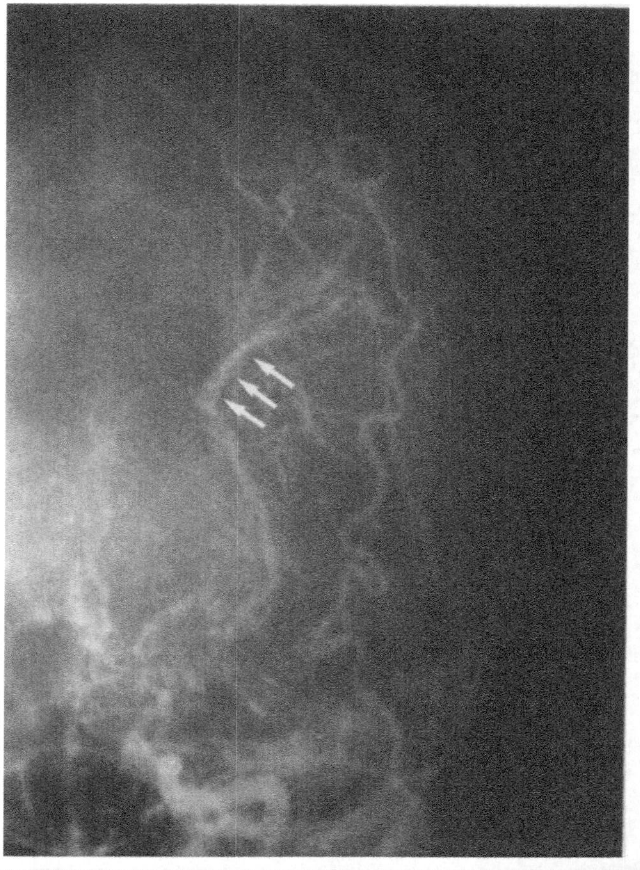

31

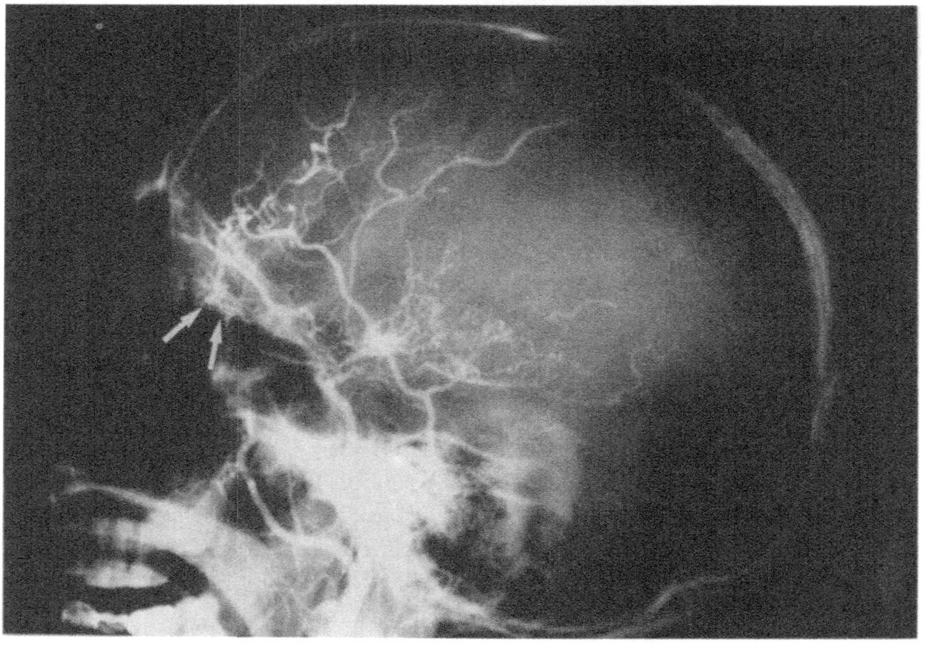

32

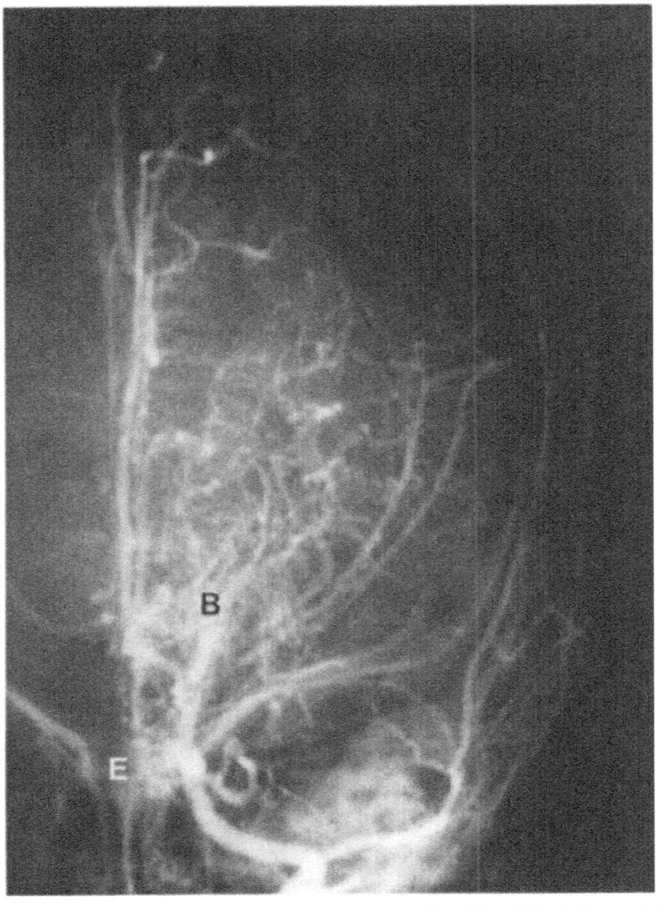

Fig. 33. A 2-year-old female case. Anteroposterior view of the left carotid angiogram at stage 3 of basal moyamoya. Basal moyamoya-like vessels which had been thought as orbital moyamoya in fact existed at the ethmoidal sinus and upper nasal meatus. Moreover, connections from these vessels to basal moyamoya were observed. *B*, basal moyamoya, *E*, ethmoidal moyamoya

◄

Fig. 31. A 56-year-old male case. Collateral pathways from the perforating branches to the medullary arteries were observed (*arrows*)

Fig. 32. A 6-year-old female case. Left carotid angiogram, lateral view. Basal moyamoya-like vessels were seen at the roof of the orbit (*arrows*)

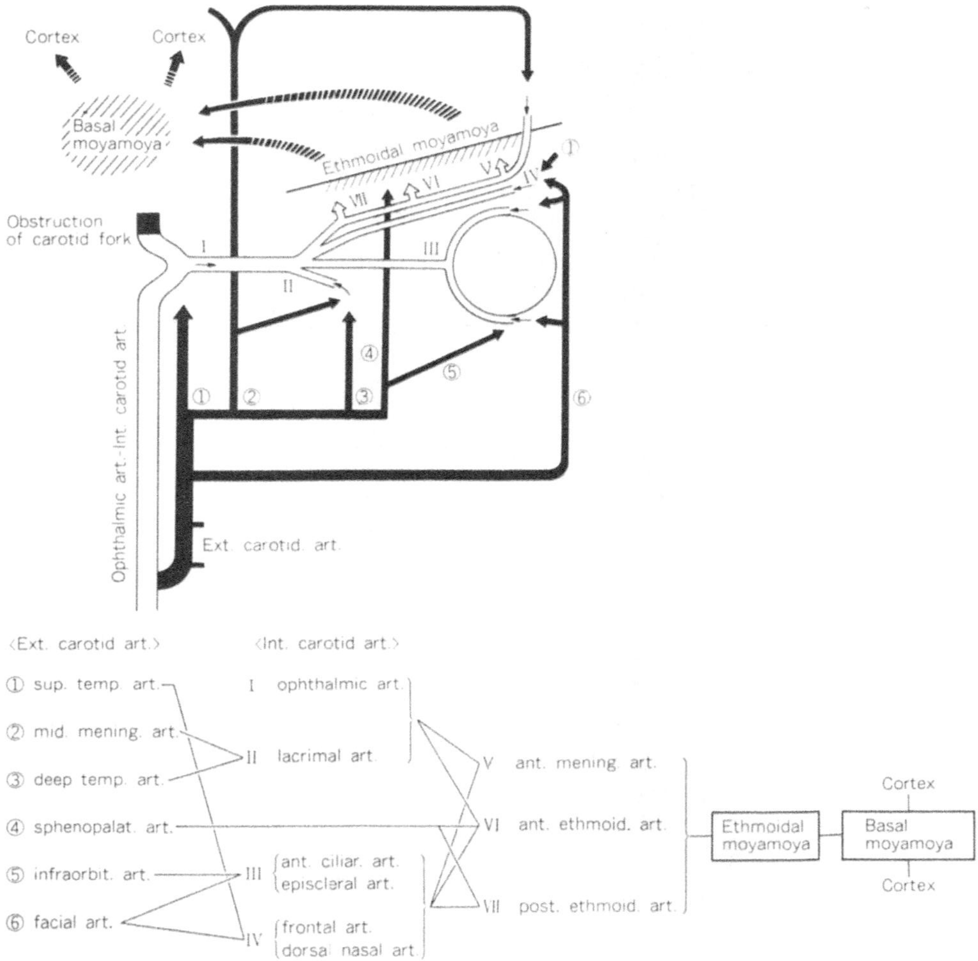

Fig. 34. The blood vessels running in and out of ethmoidal moyamoya

3.4.1 Feeding Arteries in Ethmoidal Moyamoya (Fig. 34)

Investigation of the feeding arteries in ethmoidal moyamoya was made using angiograms obtained from 38 adult cases (67 sides) and 39 juvenile cases (83 sides). Ethmoidal vessels were found to be fed from the ICA system through the arteria ophthalmica and a. ethmoidalis posterior, as well as through the a. ethmoidalis anterior. From the external carotid arterial system, the feeding arteries of ethmoidal moyamoya vessels are from the a. temporalis superficialis or from the a. facialis through the a. frontalis, a. dorsalis nasi, a. ciliares, a. episcleralis, and a. choroidea. There are also feeders to ethmoidal moyamoya through the a. ethmoidalis posterior et anterior. Feeders also arise from the a. maxillaris through the a. meningea media, a. meningea anterior, a. ethmoidalis anterior, and a. ethmoidalis posterior. Similarly, feeders are found from the a. maxillaris, a. meningea media, and a. lacrimalis through the a. ethmoidalis posterior et anterior. Finally, feeders through the a. maxillaris, a. temporalis profunda, a. lacrimalis, a. ethmoidalis posterior et anterior to ethmoidal moyamoya are found, as well as feeders from the a. maxillaris and a. sphenopalatina through the a. ethmoidalis posterior et anterior or pathways feeding directly from the so-called »ethmoidal moyamoya.«

As can be seen from the above, in ethmoidal moyamoya, vessels from various regions flow together to form a common pool, and there are also vascular connections from ethmoidal moyamoya to basal moyamoya.

In the normal state, the presence of bone and the dura mater prevents the flow of blood above the ethmoidal sinus and the wall of the upper nasal meatus. However, the olfactory nerve fibers descending from the olfactory bulb lie beneath the mucous membrane of the upper nasal cavity, and nerve endings are formed along that surface. As a clear indication that those nerves do in fact pass through the dura mater at the cranial base, the lamina cribrosa is found to have an open pore-like structure.

It is likely that the vessels passing through these pores travel with the olfactory nerve fibers and communicate with intracranial vessels. Moreover, consideration of the presence of fetal-stage vessels, such as the primitive olfactory artery, the primitive ventral ophthalmic artery, and the primitive dorsal ophthalmic artery, suggests that during a pathological state of cerebral ischemia they may recover function as arteries and work as feeders to the intracranial space from the extracranial space. Consequently, if the ischemic brain requires greater blood flow, the vessels of the ICA and ECA systems will dilatate to a maximum and expand the net-like vessels which can increase, if only slightly, the blood flow to the ethmoidal sinus and the vascular network of the mucous membrane of the upper nasal cavity. Next, travelling through a vascular system which is normally occluded almost entirely, it is probable that there is an increase of blood to the intracranial space. In summary, ethmoidal moyamoya is thought to be a state in which the vascular network of the ethmoidal sinus and the mucous membrane of the upper nasal cavity are dilatated.

3.4.2 Incidence of Ethmoidal Moyamoya and Its Correlation with Six Stages of Basal Moyamoya (Table 4)

A study was also carried out of the correlation between the various stages of basal moyamoya and the degree of ethmoidal moyamoya. In young patients it was found that, as the basal moyamoya entered a late stage, there was a tendency for the ethmoidal moyamoya to increase gradually. As the stenosis of the terminal portion of the ICA progresses, the blood supply to the base of the brain decreases, and, to

Table 4. Incidence of ethmoidal moyamoya and correlation between ethmoidal moyamoya and the stage of basal moyamoya. Ethmoidal moyamoya develops with the stage of basal moyamoya in juvenile cases but there is no correlation between the two in adult cases

	Incidence and degree of ethmoidal moyamoya	Communicating vessels between ethmoidal moyamoya and basal moyamoya	Correlation between degrees of ethmoidal moyamoya and stages of basal moyamoya: Ethmoidal moyamoya	Basal moyamoya
Juvenile cases			(−) —	stage 1 — 4
			(+) —	stage 1 — 4
39 cases	(−) — 4	(−) — 6		stage 2 — 3
83 sides	(+) — 9	(+) — 14		stage 3 — 5
	(++) — 11	(++) — 18	(++) —	stage 1 — 2
	(+++) — 59	(+++) — 45		stage 3 — 5
				stage 4 — 4
				stage 5 — 6
			(+++) —	stage 3 — 12
				stage 4 — 16
				stage 5 — 11
	95.2%	92.8%		stage 6 — 11
Adult cases			(−) —	normal or stage 1 — 7
				stage 4 — 5
38 cases 67 sides	(−) — 17	(−) — 26		stage 5 — 5
	(+) — 34	(+) — 28	(+) —	normal or stage 1 — 2
	(++) — 8	(++) — 7		stage 3 — 7
	(+++) — 8	(+++) — 6		stage 4 — 7
				stage 5 — 11
			(++) —	stage 3 — 3
				stage 4 — 6
	74.6%	61.2%	(+++) —	stage 4 — 4
				stage 5 — 5
				stage 6 — 4

that degree, blood supply to the brain from ethmoidal moyamoya vessels is thought to have increased. In fact, it has been found that in young cases, when the basal moyamoya enters stage 5, the blood flow through the basal moyamoya vessels becomes extremely slight, whereas that through the ethmoidal moyamoya increases (Figs. 35–37).

In adult cases, on the other hand, ethmoidal moyamoya could not definitely be correlated with each phase of basal moyamoya. Most such cases showed only poor development of ethmoidal moyamoya even when basal moyamoya had reached the fifth stage or gave evidence of several large collateral vessels running into the brain (Fig. 38). However, there was an exceptionally prominent growth of

Fig. 36. The same case as in Fig. 35 at stage 3 of basal moyamoya. The development of ethmoidal moyamoya is seen (*arrows*)

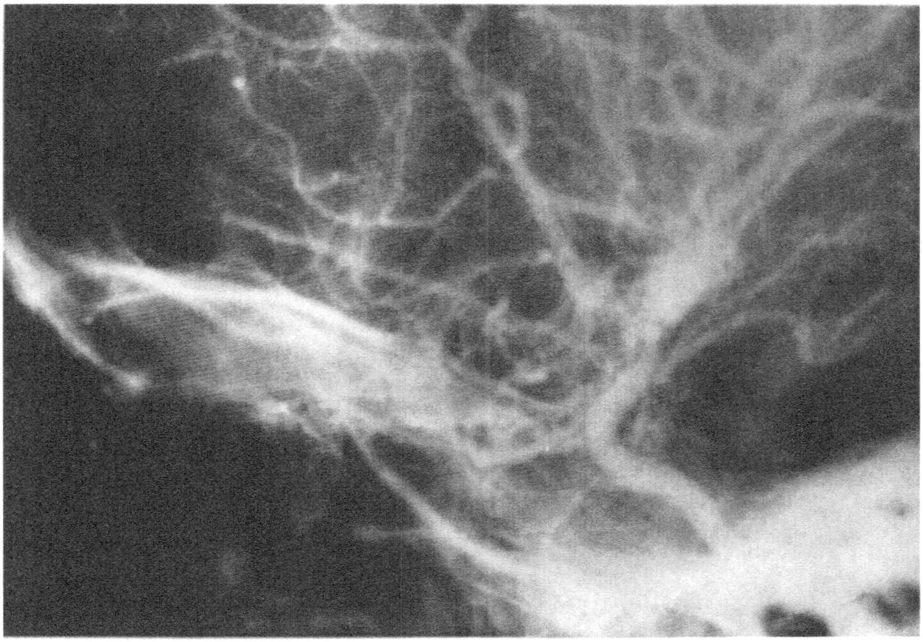

Fig. 35. The correlation between ethmoidal moyamoya and the stage of basal moyamoya in juvenile cases. No ethmoidal is seen at stage 2 of basal moyamoya

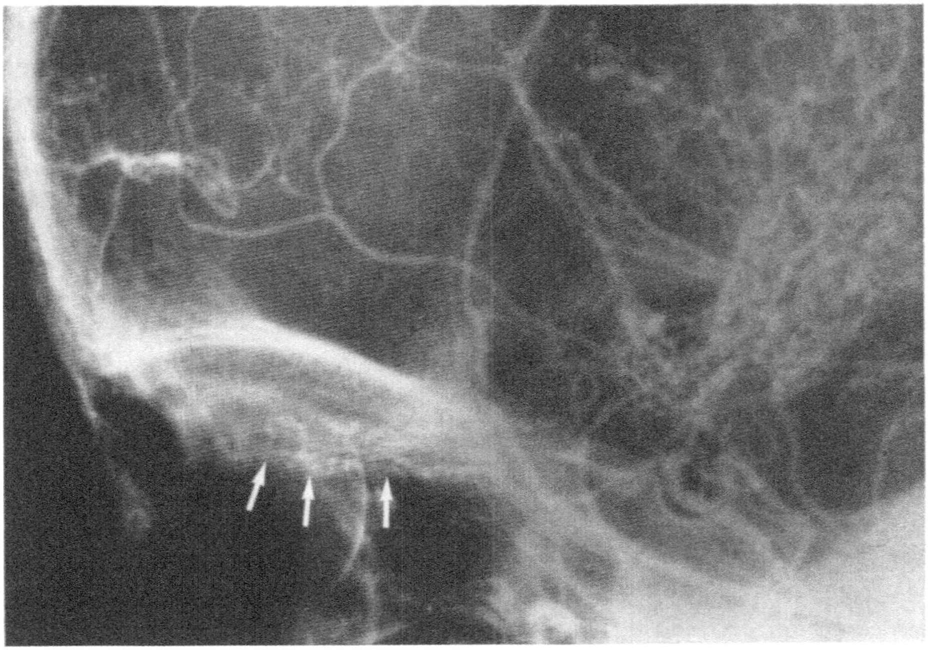

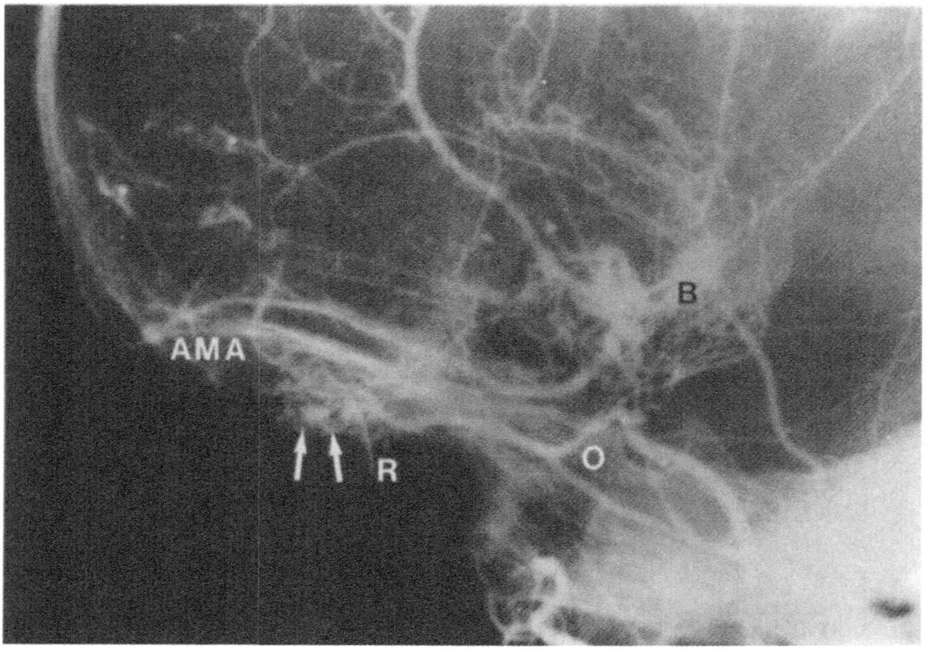

Fig. 37. The same case as in Figs. 35 and 36 at stage 4 of basal moyamoya. The ethmoidal moyamoya becomes prominent (*arrows*) and retrobulbar vascular shadow is clearly observed. *B*, basal moyamoya; *O*, ophthalmic artery; *R*, retrobulbar vascular shadow; *AMA*, anterior meningeal artery

ethmoidal moyamoya in a few patients in whom basal moyamoya was then supposed to be in the fifth or sixth stage. These features of ethmoidal moyamoya and basal moyamoya in adults were considerably different from those in the young. It seems to us that adults probably presented such an irregular and poorly developed pattern of ethmoidal moyamoya because they had already lost the ability to widen or reopen blood vessels which the young still possessed.

Since the adult patients followed up angiographically did not show, as we have already mentioned, any remarkable change in their pattern of basal moyamoya, it was supposed that the present disease in adults might have occurred at a young age and that its progression might have come to a standstill at a certain stage of the disease. If that is true, ethmoidal moyamoya, which tends to occur at a young age, must be still observable in adulthood. In fact, however, few adults have shown evidence of well-formed ethmoidal moyamoya (Fig. 39). It is consequently safer to suggest that the disease in most adult patients occurred during adulthood. Nevertheless, a few adult patients have shown evidence of well-developed ethmoidal moyamoya, so it is reasonable to suppose that the occurrence of this disease in such adult cases was in childhood, and that development of the disease process came to a standstill at a certain phase.

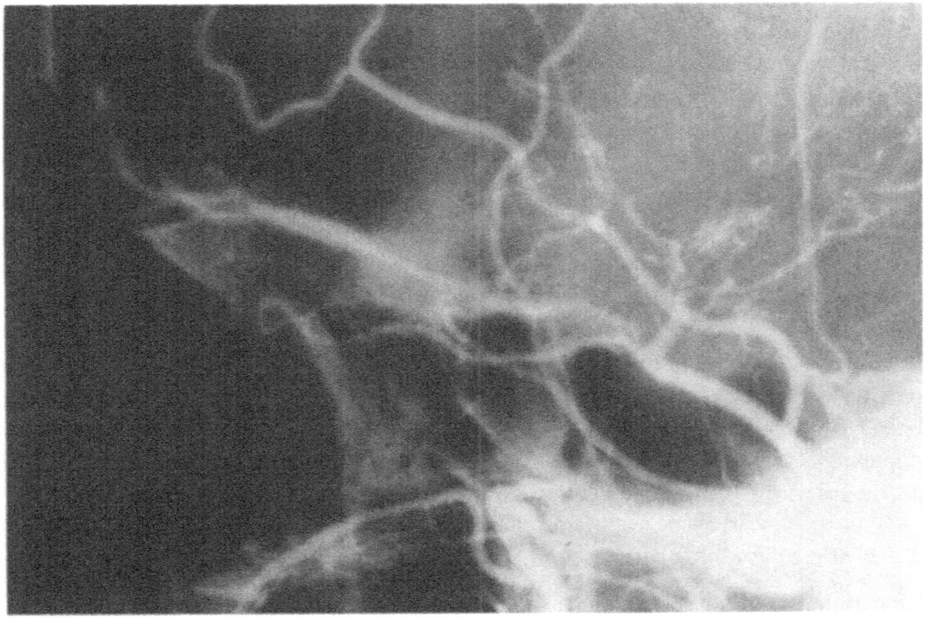

Fig. 38. A 29-year-old female case. In almost all adult cases very poor development of ethmoidal moyamoya is seen, as in this patient in spite of the progressed stage of basal moyamoya

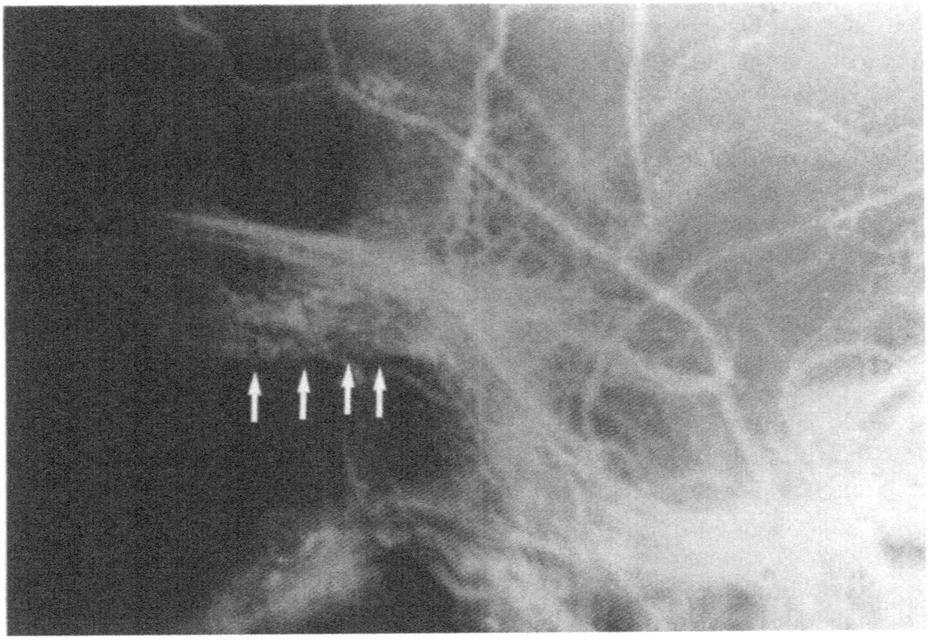

Fig. 39. A 47-year-old female case. In a few adult cases, remarkable development of ethmoidal moyamoya is seen, as in this patient (*arrows*)

3.5 Vault Moyamoya

Vault moyamoya is an abnormal network of vessels similar to the above-mentioned basal moyamoya and ethmoidal moyamoya, in which moyamoya vessels are also seen at the cranial vault. For this reason, this condition has been labeled »vault moyamoya« [41, 136]. Serial cerebral angiograms have shown that in vault moyamoya blood is supplied to the brain by means of the formation of pathways from the external carotid arterial system (Figs. 40, 41). It is thought that such vessels are collateral pathways formed by the anastomosis of the dural arteries and the pial arteries, a phenomenon also known as rete mirabile anastomosis [20, 185, 300, 319]. This dural-pial anastomosis may be residual from the fetal stage, but vault moyamoya characteristically shows a few collateral pathways at the adhesion with the surface of the brain where surface veins run beneath the dura mater and enter the venous sinus. As cerebral blood flow decreases, these vessels expand to a network and form a system of collateral pathways to the brain which is thought to be the essence of vault moyamoya.

3.5.1 Site of Vault Moyamoya and Its Feeding Arteries

Investigation of vault moyamoya was made using angiograms obtained from 39 juvenile cases (83 sides) and 38 adult cases (67 sides). The sites of vault moyamoya were fairly consistent in both juvenile and adult cases. Nine distinct sites of vault moyamoya were found in the juvenile cases. They were: a frontal pole paramedian region (FPM), a bregma paramedian region (BRM), a bregma lateral region (BRL), a parietal paramedian region (PP), a parietal lateral region (PL), a parietooccipital paramedian region (POM), a parietooccipital lateral region (POL), an occipital lateral region (OL), and a paratransverse sinus region (T) (Fig. 42). In the adult cases, vault moyamoya was seen at all but three of these sites. It was not seen at the BRL, PM, and PL regions (Fig. 43). It is possible that these three sites were not seen due to occasional deviation of the subject. Although the number of adult cases with vault moyamoya at such sites would still be small, such cases may occur. Moreover, although the feeding arteries of vault moyamoya and the arteries forming the moyamoya network differ slightly among individual cases, the same vessels are normally involved (Table 5). According to the site of the vault moyamoya, these vessels are as follows:

1. FPM: The main feeding artery is the anterior meningeal artery (AMA), but the frontal branch of the superficial temporal artery (STA) and occasionally the frontal branch of the middle meningeal artery (MMA) can also serve as feeding arteries (Fig. 44).
2. BRM: The main feeding artery is the frontal branch of the MMA, but the frontal branch of the STA and the AMA are sometimes feeding arteries to vault moyamoya in this region (Figs. 45,46).
3. BRL: The main feeding artery is the frontal branch of the MMA and feeding arteries can also include the parietal branch of the MMA (Fig. 47).

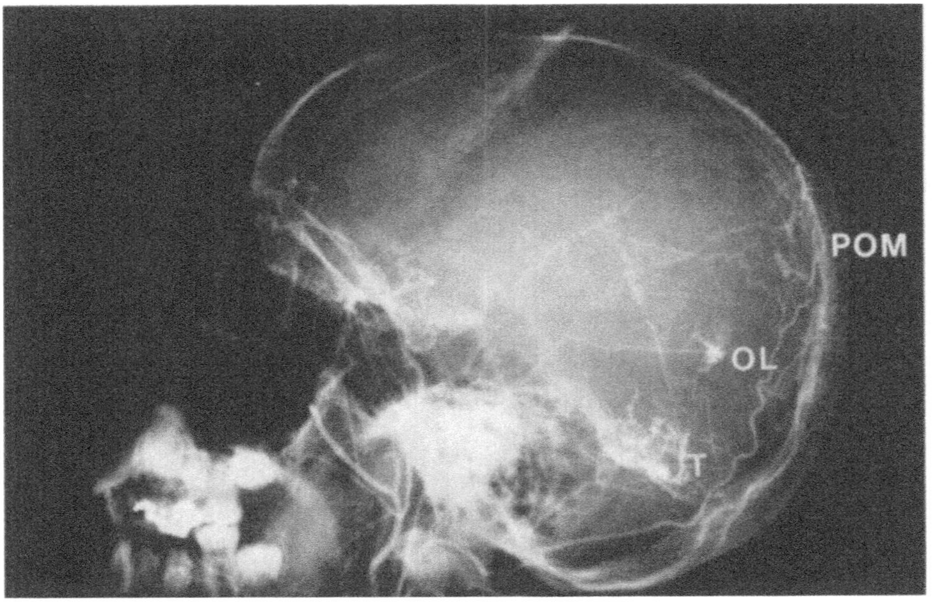

Fig. 40. Vault moyamoya. Three basal moyamoya-like vessels (vault moyamoya) are seen at the parietooccipital (*POM*), occipital (*OL*), and paratransverse sinus region (*T*)

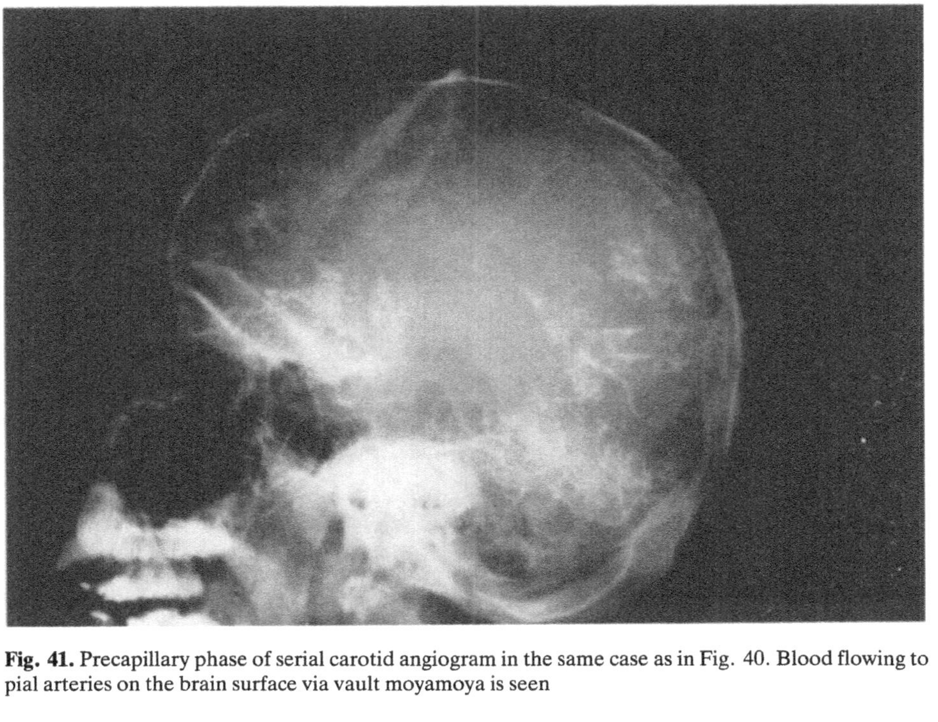

Fig. 41. Precapillary phase of serial carotid angiogram in the same case as in Fig. 40. Blood flowing to pial arteries on the brain surface via vault moyamoya is seen

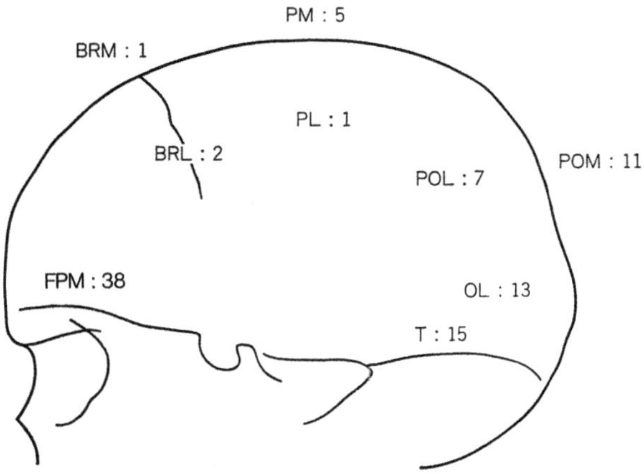

Fig. 42. Location and number of vault moyamoya in juvenile cases (89 sides in 39 cases). The incidence of vault moyamoya is higher at sites near the base of the brain, with a characteristically lower incidence as one moves away from the region. *PL*, parietal lateral region; *OL*, occipital lateral region; *T*, paratransverse sinus region; *BRL*, bregma lateral region; *PM* parietal paramedian region; *FPM*, frontal pole paramedian region; *BRM*, bregma paramedian region; *POM*, parietooccipital paramedian region; *POL*, parietooccipital lateral region

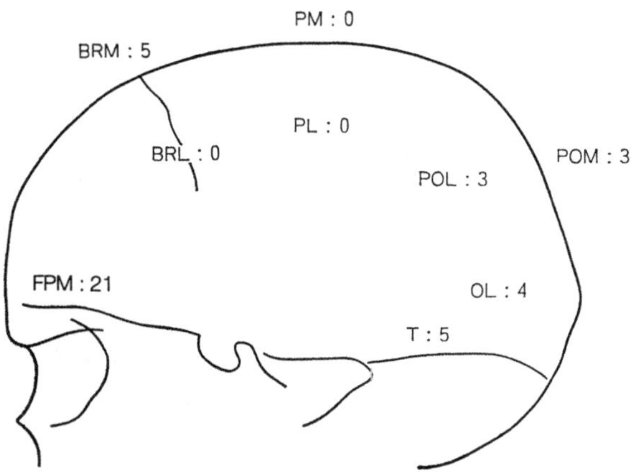

Fig. 43. Location and number of vault moyamoya in adult cases (67 sides in 38 cases). The incidence of vault moyamoya is higher at sites near the base of the brain as in children, but in adults there are apparently three sites (*BRL, PM,* and *PL*) where vault moyamoya has not been observed at all. Abbreviations as for Fig. 42

Table 5. Feeding arteries to vault moyamoya

	Feeder					
Location	AMA	MMA	PMA	TA	STA	OA
FPM	●	○f			○p	
BRM	○	●f			○p	
BRL		●f ○f				
PM	○	●f			○p	
PL		●p				
POM		●p			○p	
POL		●p				
OL		●p	○			○
T			○	●		

AMA, anterior meningeal artery; MMA, middle meningeal artery; PMA, posterior meningeal artery; TA, tentorial artery; STA, superficial temporal artery; OA, occipital artery; f, frontal branch; p, parietal branch; ●, main feeding artery; ○, accessory feeding artery

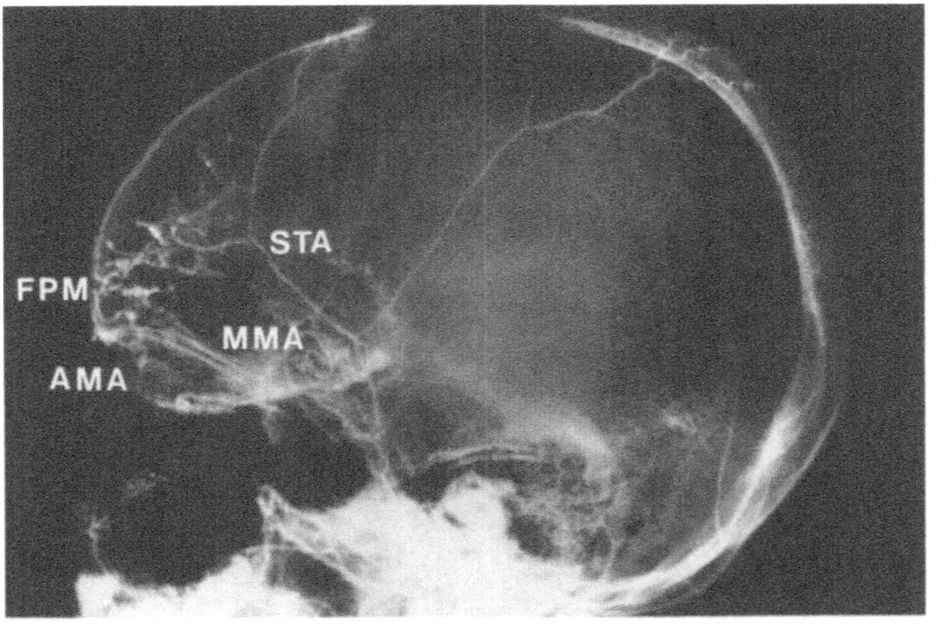

Fig. 44. Vault moyamoya at the frontal pole paramedian region (*FPM*). The main feeder is the *AMA* and feeding from the frontal branch of *STA* and *MMA* is also seen. *STA*, superficial temporal artery; *MMA*, middle meningeal artery; *AMA*, anterior meningeal artery

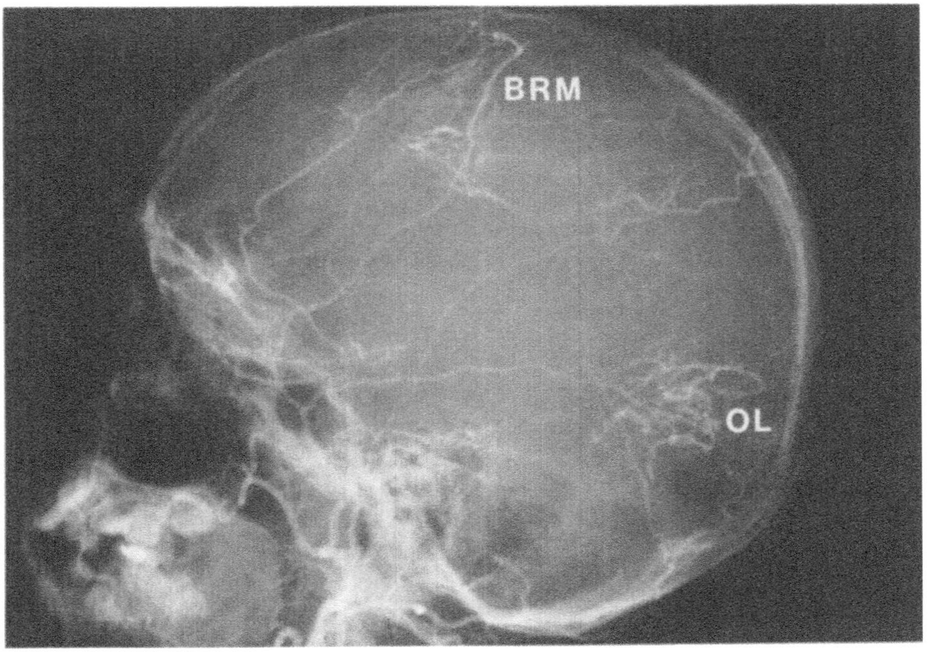

Fig. 45. Vault moyamoya at the bregma paramedian region (*BRM*) and the occipital lateral region (*OL*). Blood flowing from the *BRM* to the pericallosal artery is visualized

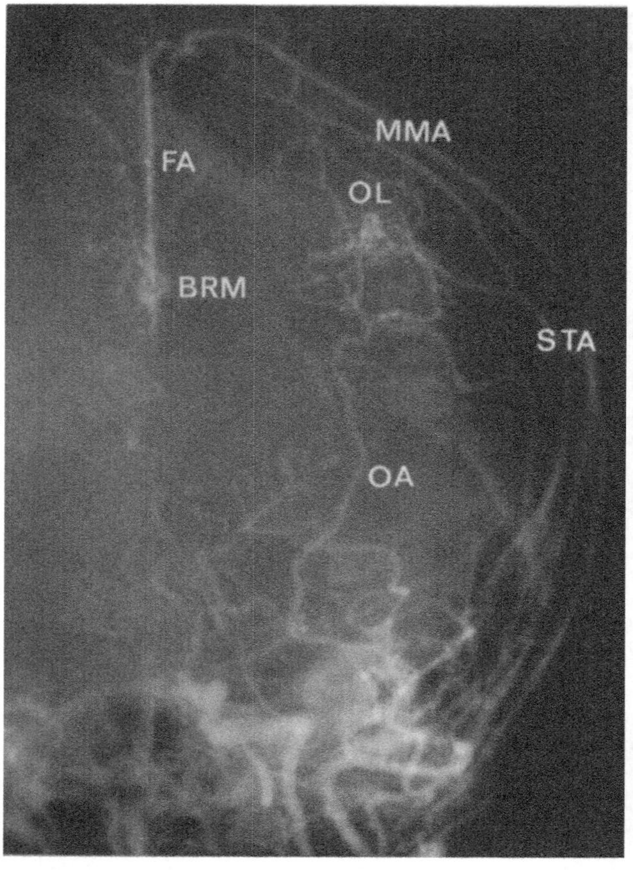

Fig. 46. Anteroposterior view of the same case as in Fig. 45. Vault moyamoya at the *BRM* and *OL*, and their feeding arteries are clearly visualized. *FA*, falx artery; *OA*, occipital artery; *BRM*, bregma paramedian region; *OL*, occipital lateral region; *MMA*, middle meningeal artery; *STA*, superficial temporal artery

4. PM: The parietal branch of the MMA is the main feeding artery. Feeders can also include the parietal branch of the STA and the AMA (Figs. 47,48).
5. PL: The parietal branch of the MMA is the main feeder.
6. POM: The parietal branch of the MMA is the main feeder, with blood also flowing from the parietal branch of the STA (Fig. 47).
7. POL: The parietal branch of the MMA is the main feeding artery (Fig. 49).
8. OL: The main feeder is the parietal branch of the MMA, with the moyamoya network also being fed by the occipital artery (OA) and sometimes the posterior meningeal artery (PMA) (Figs. 45,46).
9. T: The tentorial artery (TA) is the main feeder, while blood also flows through the PMA (Fig. 50).

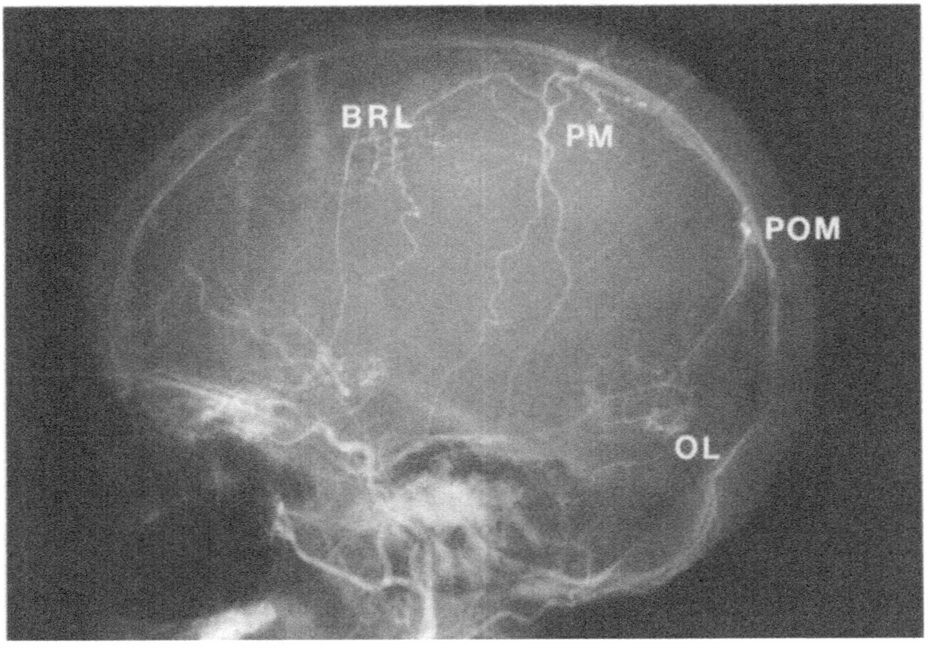

Fig. 47. Vault moyamoya at the bregma lateral region (*BRL*), the parietal paramedian region (*PM*), the parietooccipital paramedian region (*POM*), and the occipital lateral region (*OL*)

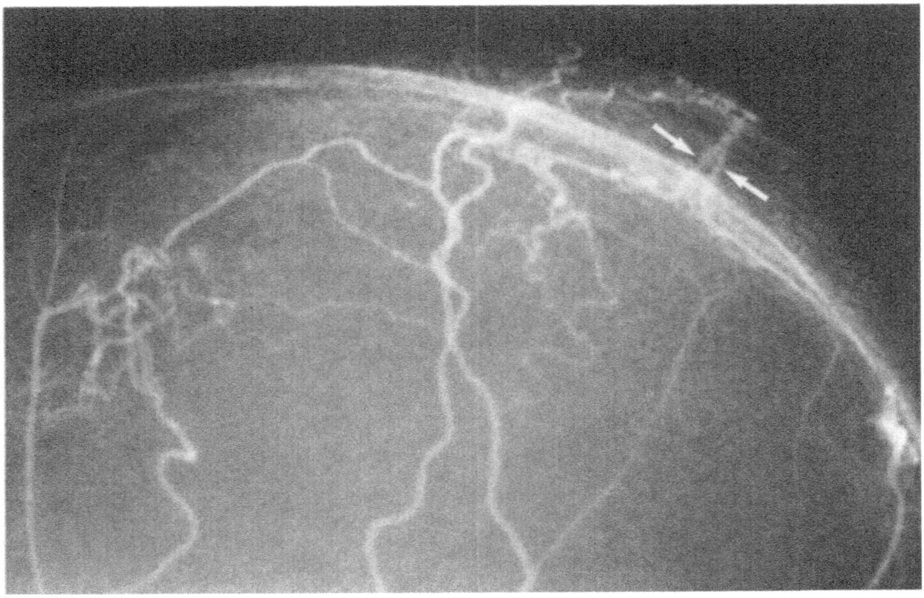

Fig. 48. Vault moyamoya at the parietal paramedian region in the same case as in Fig. 47. Anastomoses between the superficial temporal artery and middle meningeal artery are seen (*arrows*)

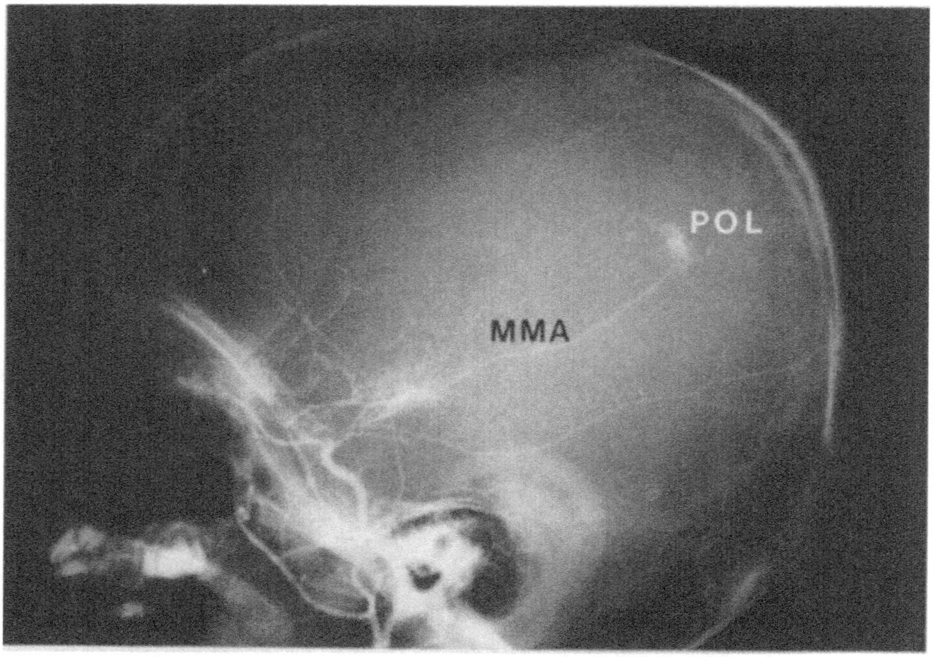

Fig. 49. Vault moyamoya at the parietooccipital lateral region (*POL*), *MMA*, middle meningeal artery

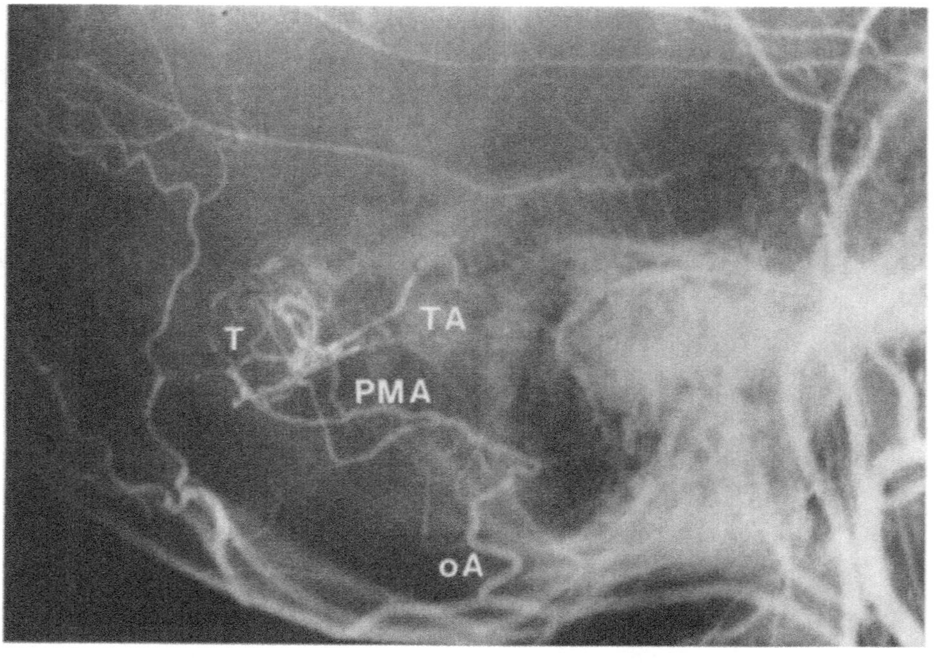

Fig. 50. Vault moyamoya at the paratransverse sinus region (*T*). *TA*, tentorial artery; *PMA*, posterior meningeal artery; *OA*, occipital artery

Among those cases of vault moyamoya in a paramedian location, there were some in which blood flowed to the pial arteries from the falx or tentorium, but the large majority of these cases showed blood flow from the vault moyamoya directly to the pial arteries.

3.5.2 Incidence of Vault Moyamoya at Various Sites and Its Correlation with the Six Stages of Basal Moyamoya (Tables 6, 7, Figs. 42,43)

Investigation of the incidence of vault moyamoya according to site in the juvenile cases showed that by far the most common site was FPM (41%), followed by T and OL, whereas in the adult cases FPM was the most common (51%) followed byT, BRM, and OL. Although there were some differences between the juvenile and adult groups, the incidence was higher at sites near the base of the brain, with a characteristically lower incidence as one moved away from the region.

This feature of vault moyamoya is thought to reflect the physiological response to cerebral blood insufficiency at sites which are close to the terminal portion of the ICA, where vascular stenosis and occlusion are present. In other words, the collateral circulation is shunted over the shortest possible distance. Rather than

Table 6. Vault moyamoya in children

Stage of basal moyamoya	No. of CAG side	Number of vault moyamoya									No. appearing per one side
		FPM	BRM	BRL	PM	PL	POM	POL	OL	T	
I	10										0(0/10)
II	3										0(0/3)
III	31	11				1	1	1		2	0.5(15/31)
IV	21	13		1			5	1	3	6	1.4(30/21)
V	16	13		1	3		5	3	9	6	2.5(40/16)
VI	2	1	1		2			2	1	1	4.0 (8/2)
Total	83	38	1	2	5	1	11	7	13	15	1.1(93/83)

FPM, frontal pole paramedian; BRM, bregma paramedian; BRL, bregma lateral; PM, parietal paramedian; PL, parietal lateral; POM, parietooccipital paramedian; POL, parietooccipital lateral; OL, occipital lateral; T, paratransverse sinus

Table 7. Vault moyamoya in adults

Stage of basal moyamoya	No. of CAG side	Number of vault moyamoya									No. appearing per one side
		FPM	BRM	BRL	PM	PL	POM	POL	OL	T	
I	7										0(0/7)
II	0										
III	2										0(0/2)
IV	24	8	2				1	1	3	1	0.7(16/24)
V	30	10	1				1	2		1	0.5(15/30)
VI	4	3	2				1		1	3	2.5(10/4)
Total	77	21	5	0	0	0	3	3	4	5	0.6(41/67)

Abbreviations as for Table 6

developing from sites which are remote from the stenosis or occlusion, the collateral pathways develop from neighboring sites. The nature and frequency of appearance of the moyamoya vessels seem therefore to obey this principle of formation of collateral pathways.

As a result, it can be seen that vault moyamoya is found with a high incidence at sites near the base of the brain. Blood is thought to be supplied to the base of the frontal lobe from ethmoidal moyamoya, to the frontal poles from vault moyamoya of the FPM region, to the base of the occipital lobe from moyamoya of the T region, and to the lateral aspects of the occipital lobe from moyamoya of the OL region.

Since there are two blood supply pathways leading to both the frontal lobe and the occipital lobe, it is difficult to understand why no collateral pathways are found from the middle fossa to the temporal lobe. Theoretically, there is a strong possibility that collateral pathways from the middle fossa would be present, but largely because of the complexity of the base of the cranium as seen in plain skull X-ray images they cannot be identified. The presence of such collateral pathways may perhaps be demonstrated by »subtraction« of the angiographical images obtained from the base of the skull and other such manipulations.

With regard to the correlation between vault moyamoya and basal moyamoya, it was found that there was no vault moyamoya at stage 1 or stage 2 in the child group, but moyamoya was more frequently found, the later the stage (stages 3–6). That is, the degree to which the stenosis of the terminal portion of the ICA had progressed, and consequently the degree to which blood supply to the brain was reduced, is reflected in the incidence of vault moyamoya.

In the adult cases, the vessels which formed vault moyamoya were larger and coarser and there were subtle differences between the juvenile and adult disease states. That is, there was no vault moyamoya at stages 1, 2, or 3 and only a few cases at stages 4 or 5. There were, however, twice as many at stage 6 at as stage 4 or 5. No strong correlation, though, was seen between the stage and incidence of vault moyamoya. In the adult cases where sequential follow-up angiography was performed, there were virtually no changes in the shape or site of either vault moyamoya or basal moyamoya, and thus far we have not experienced a single case in which vault moyamoya appeared during the period of follow-up.

The problem of when vault moyamoya arose in these adult cases still remains. The vault moyamoya seen in adults may be vault moyamoya that formed in childhood and remained more or less unchanged until adulthood, but there is clearly less vault moyamoya among adults and there are apparently three sites (BRL, PM, and PL) where the moyamoya vessel has not been observed at all. It cannot therefore be asserted that in all adult moyamoya cases vault moyamoya develops in childhood and remains dormant until adulthood. Particularly in light of the fact that there are some adult cases which are known to have developed vault moyamoya in adulthood, it is possible that in these patients vault moyamoya did not easily arise because of a low capacity to form collateral pathways.

3.6 Cerebral Angiograms Taken After Hyperventilation

Details will be provided in Chap. 4 on the EEG, but it is currently thought that a »re-buildup phenomenon« [9, 135, 269] in the EEG following hyperventilation is unique to this disease. It remains unclear precisely what causes this phenomenon, but we have recently obtained some interesting angiographical findings following hyperventilation in a 17-year-old girl with this disease (Fig. 51). However, it is unknown now whether or not this unusual angiographical image is in any way characteristic of moyamoya disease or unique to this particular case.

A

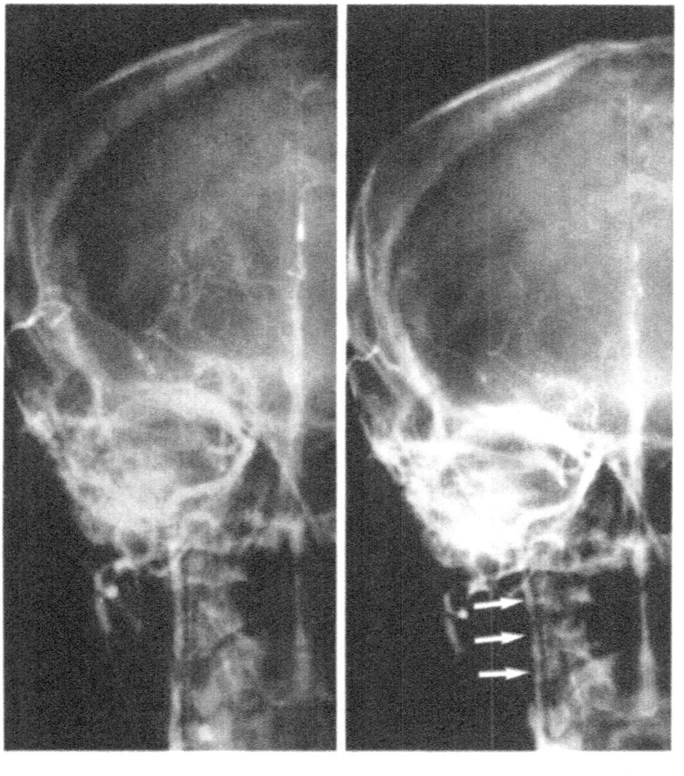

B

Fig. 51 A, B. A 17-year-old female case. Right carotid angiogram before **A** and 1 min after **B** hyperventilation. The »re-buildup phenomenon« was found on EEG from 1 min after the cessation of hyperventilation for 3 min in this patient. Right carotid angiogram taken after hyperventilation (*right*) showed obvious narrowing of the neck portion of the internal carotid artery (*arrows*) and reduction of basal moyamoya

3.7 Summary

Based upon angiographical findings in moyamoya disease, the characteristic features of basal moyamoya, ethmoidal moyamoya, and vault moyamoya have been discussed. All these forms of moyamoya are thought to be collateral pathways appearing in response to cerebral blood flow insufficiency which is caused by stenosis of the terminal portions of the internal carotid arteries bilaterally. These angiographical findings suggest that moyamoya vessels are a physiological response of the vascular system to maintain sufficient blood flow to the brain.

4 Mechanisms of Symptomatic Occurrence

4.1 Introduction

The most characteristic symptom of moyamoya disease in children is repeated transient ischemic attacks (TIA), whereas in adults it is usually intracranial hemorrhage of sudden onset. Since the symptomatology of moyamoya disease has been considered previously in detail [12, 200, 206, 210], discussion in this chapter will focus on the causal mechanisms of symptoms in moyamoya disease.

4.2 Mechanism of TIA in Children (Fig. 52)

Moyamoya disease is found to progress through six stages, as judged by the dynamic changes seen in carotid angiograms (see Chap. 3). The perforating branches from the A_1 and M_1 portions near the carotid fork become occluded on the left or right, and ischemic symptoms arise at those areas of the brain which are normally fed by these arteries. In juvenile cases, however, collateral pathways are easily formed [129], and the blood supply to those areas is quickly restored over different vascular routes. Consequently, the symptoms of brain ischemia soon disappear. In this way, transient motor disturbances, such as right or left hemiparesis, are thought to arise. Similarly, short-term disturbances of consciousness may also occur.

In stage 3, it is known that the individual vessels of the moyamoya vessels are thick and clearly visible. At this stage, the fact that occlusion of perforating branches is slight and remaining perforating branches are found is thought to demonstrate that these vessels are still functioning as collateral pathways.

In stage 4, since the perforating branches become occluded as far as the peripheral portions of A_1 and M_1, gradually the moyamoya vessels become occluded and connot be individually detected on angiography. At this time, however, the collateral pathways of ethmoidal moyamoya from the external carotid and basilar arterial systems become dominant. The occluded perforating branches disappear on the angiograms, so that the frequency of TIA-like symptoms decreases.

In stage 5, the extent of the basal moyamoya vessels further decreases and, finally, in stage 6 the moyamoya vessels from the anterior cerebral circulatory system disappear entirely. In this stage, the brain is perfused solely by the

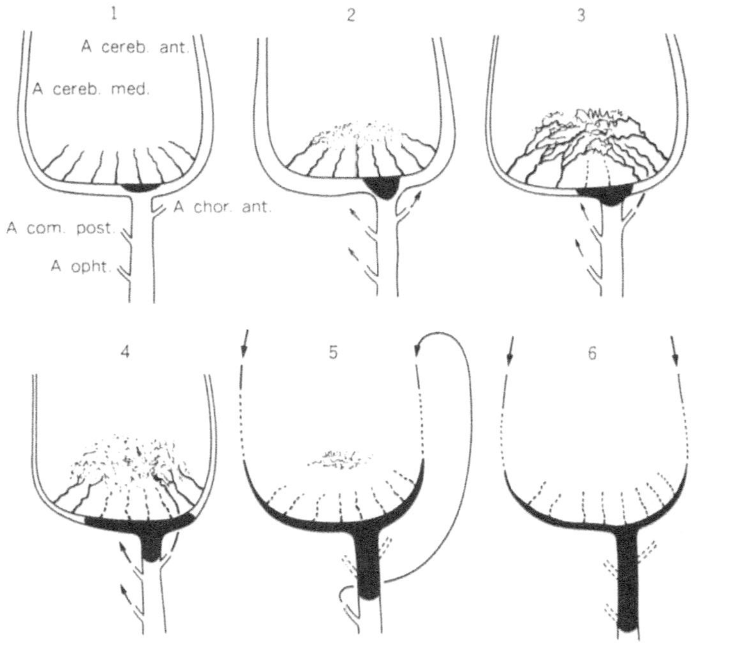

Fig. 52. Mechanism of TIA-like attacks in children. During the period from stage *1* to stage *4*, transient ischemic symptoms appear repeatedly in accordance with obstruction of perforating arteries one after another. No more transient ischemic symptoms occur in stages *5* and *6*, but mental handicap remains

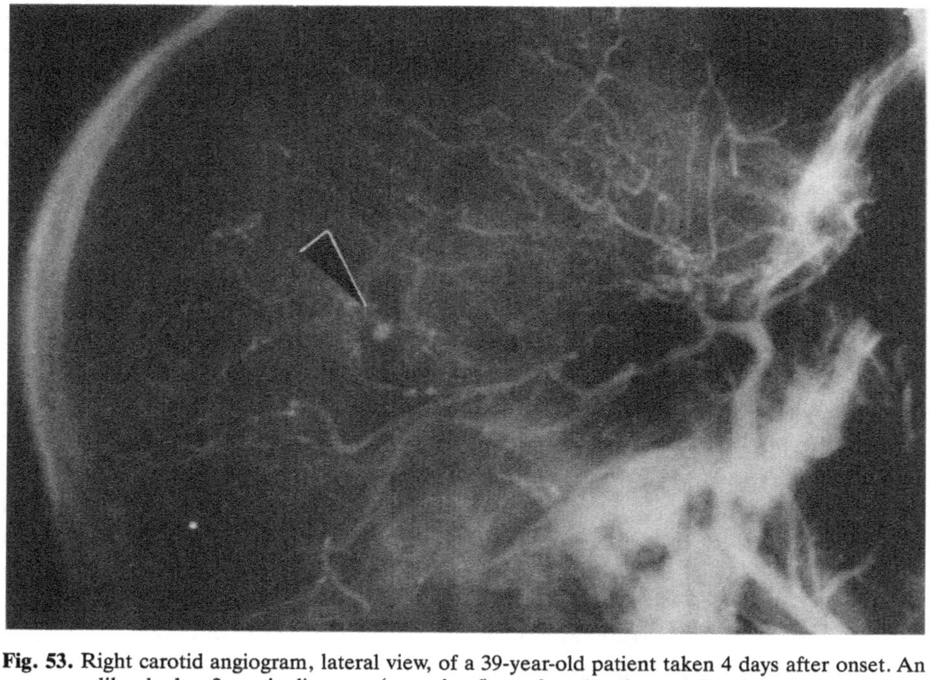

Fig. 53. Right carotid angiogram, lateral view, of a 39-year-old patient taken 4 days after onset. An aneurysm-like shadow 3 mm in diameter (*arrowhead*) was found at the peripheral portion of the right posterior choroidal artery and remained until the precapillary phase

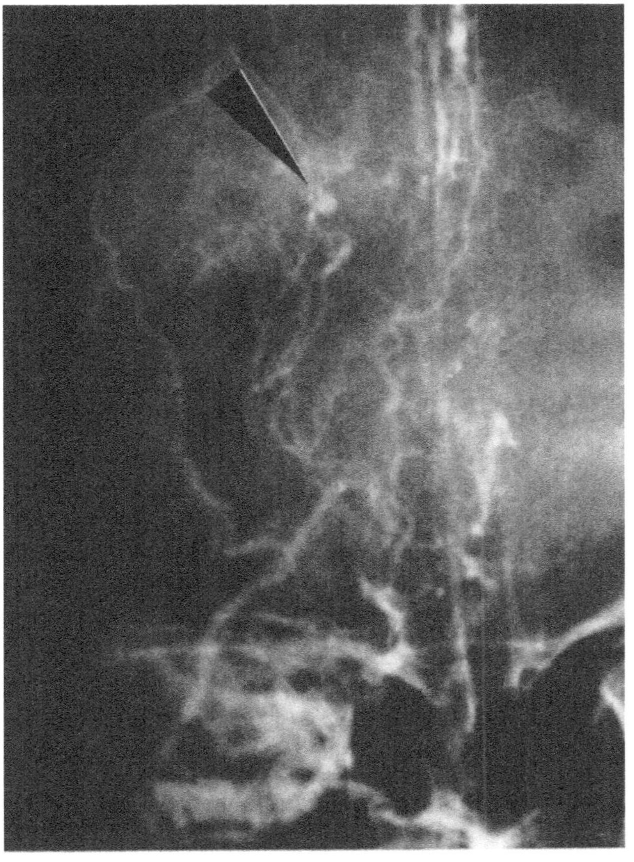

Fig. 54. The anteroposterior view of the right carotid angiogram of the same patient as in Fig. 53. An aneurysm-like shadow similar to one on the lateral view was observed at the upper lateral edge of the lateral ventricle at about 30 mm from the midline

collateral pathways from the external carotid and basilar arterial systems. By this time, all TIA-like symptoms have already disappeared, but symptoms of chronic cerebral ischemia, such as visual field defects, motor and sensory paresis, and mental retardation are apparent. It is of great interest, however, that among such cases, there are patients leading normal lives with almost no deficits of any kind.

Nevertheless, as seen during clinical examination, hyperventilation easily brings about signs of cerebral ischemia. Since cerebral circulation significantly decreases during hyperventilation [224], if cerebral blood flow at an area which tends to be slightly ischemic falls below a certain critical point, it is thought that this well induce the onset of various symptoms. Conversely, by bringing the hyperventilation to a halt, blood flow will rise above the critical point and symptoms are likely to disappear.

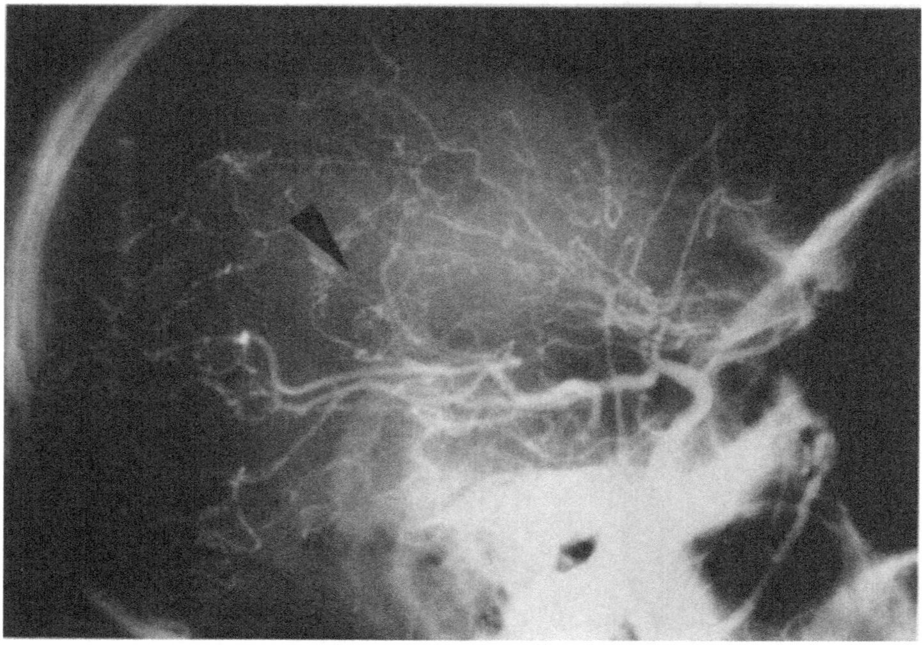

Fig. 55. Right carotid angiogram of the same patient as in Fig. 53 taken 2 months after onset. The aneurysm-like shadow at the peripheral portion of the right posterior choroidal artery had disappeared (*arrowhead*)

4.3 Mechanism of Onset of Symptoms Due to Intracranial Hemorrhage in Adults

Until recently, it has been thought that the mechanism of intracranial hemorrhage in adult cases of moyamoya disease was simply subarachnoid hemorrhage due to rupture of moyamoya vessels at the base of the brain [159, 176, 196]. Since, in most cases, patients have suffered from severe headache, their lumbar punctures showing bloody CSF without focal signs, such as hemiparesis, it has been assumed that the hemorrhage is simply a form of subarachnoid hemorrhage. The cause of the hemorrhage has been thought to lie in the rupture of the fine and easily damaged moyamoya vessels at the base of the brain. On the contrary, however, it is now believed that, for various reasons discussed below, the hemorrhage is not subarachnoid. Rather, many such cases are found to have intracerebral hemorrhage near the ventricles or to have intraventricular hemorrhage [132, 133, 296]. Consequently, even when there is intraventricular hemorrhage, the clinical manifestations are only bloody CSF and severe headache without focal signs. Therefore, the condition can easily be mistaken for subarachnoid hemorrhage. Nonetheless, there are occasionally cases of moyamoya disease with genuine saccular aneurysms [28, 131, 134], which result in genuine subarachnoid

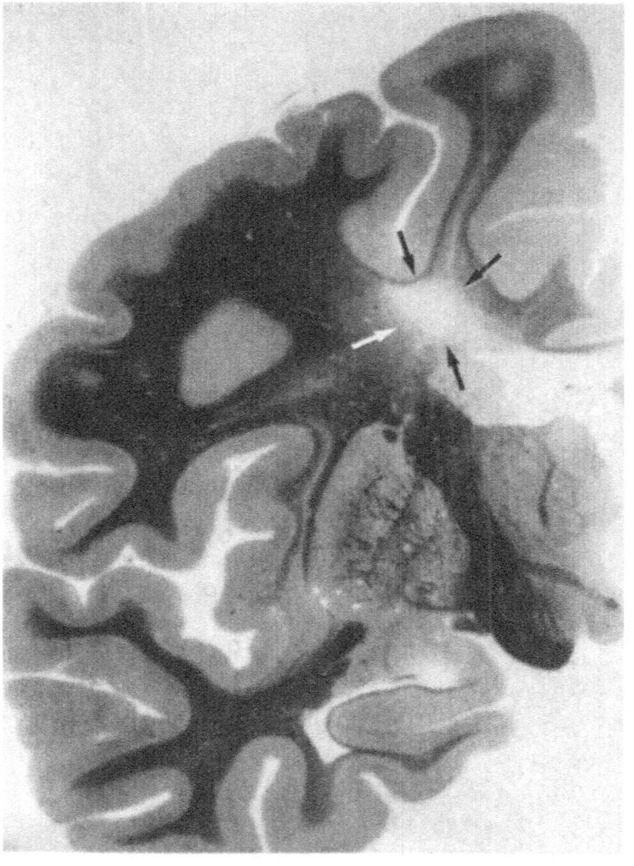

Fig. 56. Autopsied brain specimen of a 23-year-old female suffering from aortic arc syndrome. Focal softening of the brain around the upper lateral wall of the lateral ventricle is seen (*arrows*). Courtesy of Dr. Fukazawa, Research Institute of Brain and Blood Vessels, Akita, Japan)

hemorrhage. Of particular interest here is the fact that a relatively large number of the aneurysms found in association with moyamoya disease are aneurysms of the vertebrobasilar system [96, 134, 296].

4.3.1 Mechanism of Intracerebral and Intraventricular Hemorrhage

In three adult cases with onset of symptoms like those found in subarachnoid hemorrhage, we have found round aneurysm-like shadows at the peripheral portion of the lateral posterior choroidal artery (Fig. 53). In an anteroposterior view, similar shadows were seen about 30 mm from the midline at the upper lateral wall of the lateral ventricle (Fig. 54).

Follow-up angiography in these patients showed complete disappearance of the aneurysm-like shadow in all three cases (Fig. 55). Judging from the site of

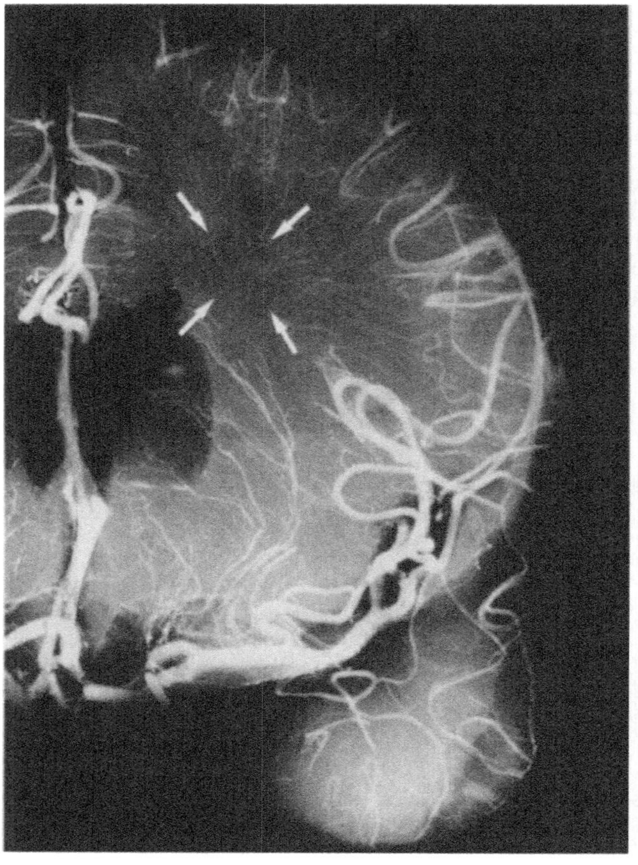

Fig. 57. Microangiogram of the autopsied brain of a 60-year-old female. The sparsest arterial distribution is recognized at the region of the upper lateral wall of the lateral ventricle (*arrows*)

these shadows at the upper lateral wall of the lateral ventricle in all three cases, these cases are thought not to have been cases of genuine cerebral aneurysms but, rather, ones in which a small pool with blood clots formed in the brain due to the rupture of a small artery at that site. That is, we believe these cases to have been »pseudoaneurysms« [98, 131, 132, 230, 317, 344] and these sites were simply the bleeding points.

It is known that an ischemic focus can easily form at the upper lateral wall of the lateral ventricles due to a circulatory disturbance, such as is found in pulseless diseases (Fig. 56). Moreover, microangiographical studies have shown that this region is that with the sparsest arterial distribution in the entire brain [133] (Fig. 57). Consequently, the capacity for developing collateral circulation is particularly poor in this region and an infarctic area is likely to form due to a chronic ischemic

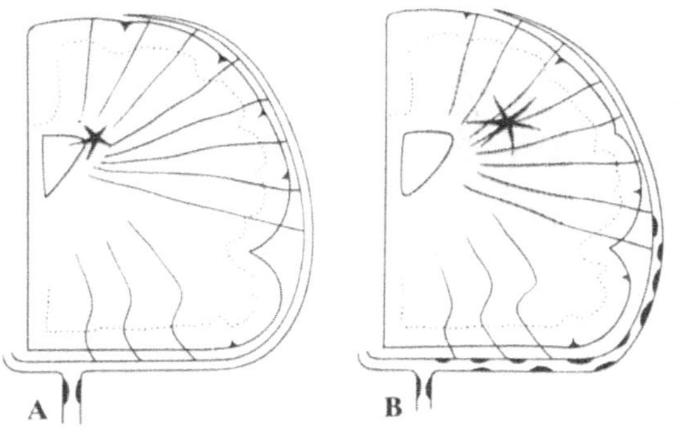

Fig. 58 A, B. Grade of cerebral circulatory insufficiency and site of hemorrhage. **A** Mild cerebral circulatory insufficiency. Small infarctic lesion of the medulla around the wall of the lateral ventricle. The hemorrhage from this lesion ruptures to the nearby ventricle. **B** Severe cerebral circulatory insufficiency. The infarctic area spreads and hemorrhage might occur from anywhere in this area. If massive bleeding occurs in the center of this lesion, hematoma will rupture to the ventricle

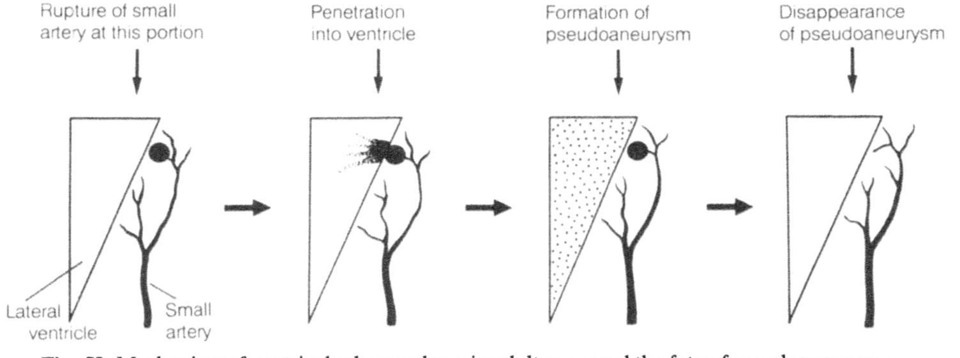

Fig. 59. Mechanism of ventricular hemorrhage in adult cases and the fate of pseudoaneurysm

state. It has also been found that collateral pathways from basal moyamoya vessels expand into this region, extending toward the cortex (Fig. 31). The weakened walls of small arteries in that region may then rupture, due to a rise in blood pressure and, depending upon the direction of the hemorrhage, either intracerebral hemorrhage or intraventricular hemorrhage will occur (Fig. 58). Moreover, aneurysm-like shadows, which are thought to be small pockets within the brain rather than genuine aneurysms, are likely to be absorbed and disappear (Fig. 59).

It is thought that the most frequent site of such pseudoaneurysms is near the paralateral wall of the lateral ventricle, but similar aneurysm-like shadows have been reported at other locations as well. It is likely that these other locations are also near the ventricular walls.

Since the introduction of CT scanning, many researchers have reported experiences of cases of intraventricular hemorrhage following intracerebral hemorrhage at the paralateral ventricular wall, which ultimately ruptures into the ventricle itself (Fig. 60). Such findings are also indicative of the mechanism mentioned above.

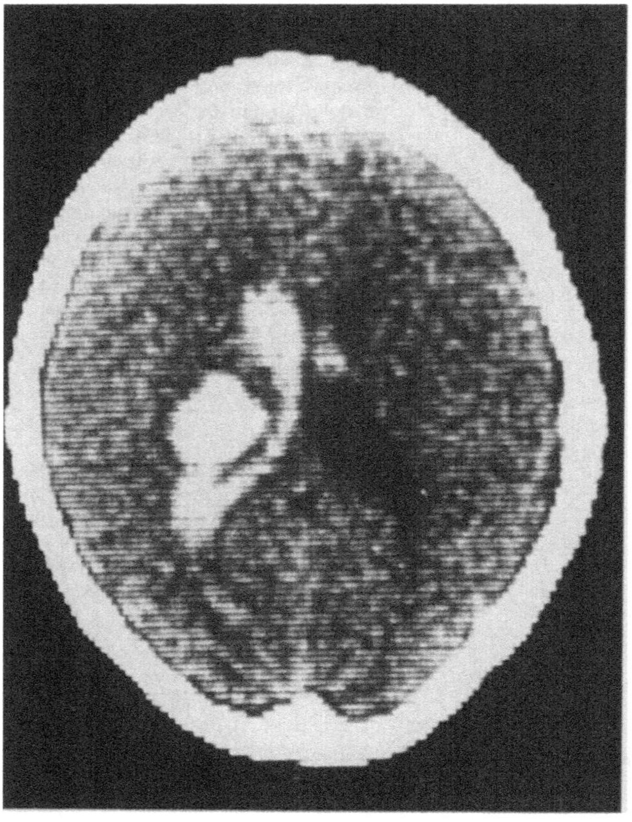

Fig. 60. Computerized tomographic scan in an adult case just after onset. Intracerebral hematoma near to the lateral ventricle ruptured to the lateral ventricle to form the ventricular hematoma

4.3.2 Onset of Symptoms in Moyamoya Disease Associated with Ruptured Saccular Aneurysms

Reports of moyamoya disease associated with ruptured cerebral aneurysms are not uncommon [1, 131, 132, 134, 228, 246] and the site of genuine saccular aneurysms in such cases is most frequently the vertebrobasilar arterial system [131, 134, 139, 183, 191, 192] (Fig. 61).

Although it is possible that aneurysms in that region could be present prior to the development of moyamoya disease, it is also possible that moyamoya disease is itself an important causal factor in the development of such aneurysms. In such a lesion, blood flow through the internal carotid arterial system gradually decreases and, simultaneously, the flow through the external carotid and vertebrobasilar arterial system increases. The pressure on the arterial walls of these latter systems is thought to increase proportionally. Therefore, if there were a congenital defect or weak point in the muscular layer of the media of the basilar

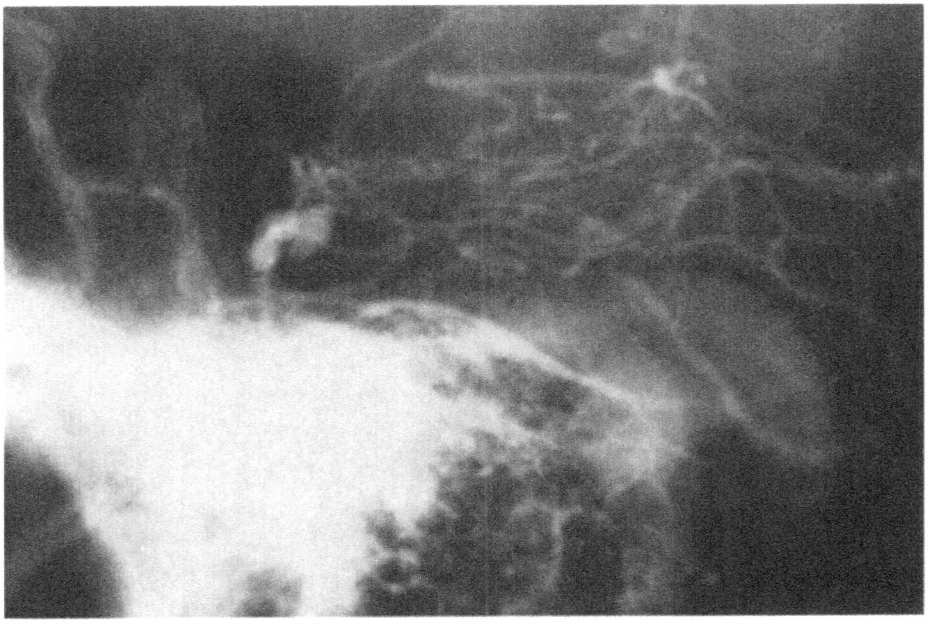

Fig. 61. Left vertebral angiogram, lateral view, of a 42-year-old male who suffered from subarachnoid hemorrhage. Two aneurysms at the basilar top were observed

arterial system, a rise in blood pressure could result in the formation of an aneurysm and its subsequent rupture.

In light of the fact that reports of moyamoya disease with aneurysms of the basilar arterial system are relatively numerous, the above mechanism may be responsible. It should be noted, however, that, although rare, there are also reports of moyamoya disease with aneurysms of the internal carotid arterial system. Aneurysms of the anterior choroidal artery are likely to be similar in nature to those of the posterior choroideal artery discussed above, but there are also reports of aneurysms of the internal carotid artery itself. In such cases, it is impossible to determine whether the aneurysm has developed as a result of moyamoya disease or has arisen by chance in association with moyamoya disease.

Finally, there are also cases in which an aneurysm ruptures and is followed by the occurrence of cerebral angiospasm in which the subsequent disturbances of blood flow cause the appearance of a fine network of collateral pathways quite similar to the network of moyamoya vessels [315]. The majority of such cases, however, show transient vascular changes; once the cerebral angiospasm has subsided, the moyamoya vessels disappear. Yet, it should be said that if an organic change is brought about by the angiospasms, it may be that moyamoya vessels remain permanently. In such cases, it would not be surprising to find an aneurysm in the internal carotid arterial system, although this would not then be considered as genuine moyamoya disease.

4.4 Summary

The mechanism involved in the occurrence of transient ischemic attack-like symptoms in juvenile cases of moyamoya disease and in the occurrence of intracranial hemorrhage in adult cases are discussed in the light of pathological findings, cerebral angiographical findings, and known cerebral hemodynamics.

5 Electroencephalography

5.1 Introduction

Yoshii and Kudo [354, 355] were the first to point out the appearance of slow waves due to hyperventilation in the electroencephalograms (EEG) of juvenile cases of moyamoya disease. Such slow waves, however, subsequently came to be considered simply as a buildup phenomenon or its prolongation [116, 348]. In other reports [212, 354] it was considered to be merely a nonspecific response seen during cerebral circulatory insufficiency. Since those early studies, we have reported on the monorhythmic posterior slow waves seen in juvenile moyamoya disease and have found that the changes seen after hyperventilation are not merely buildup or its prolongation, but that subsequent to the disappearance of slow waves. Moreover, the shape of the waves seen in moyamoya disease is distinct from such buildup, which we have labeled »re-buildup.« These EEG findings are characteristic of juvenile moyamoya disease and we have frequently emphasized the fact that EEG examination is an effective means of screening for juvenile moyamoya disease [8, 9, 74, 135, 269].

In this chapter the EEG findings in both juvenile and adult moyamoya disease based upon our clinical experiences are discussed, and evoked potential work in this disease is briefly mentioned.

5.2 Electrical Activity of the Brain in Juvenile Moyamoya Disease

Investigation of the electrical activity of the brain in 34 cases of juvenile moyamoya disease was undertaken. In general, it was found that the electrical activity in juvenile cases is severely abnormal in comparison with the EEGs recorded from adult cases (Table 8). These abnormalities are characteristically of two types: slow waves at rest and abnormal EEG changes due to hyperventilation.

5.2.1 Slow Waves at Rest

5.2.1.1 Posterior Slow Waves (P-slow)

P-slow waves are high-voltage slow waves predominantly seen in the occipital region and over the frontal lobe (Fig. 62). The frequency of such slow waves is

Table 8. Electroencephalographic findings in our cases: comparison between juvenile and adult cases (Hiraga [74]). In general, severer abnormalities in EEG are detected in juvenile than in adult cases

	Juvenile cases	Adult cases
High abnormal	5	
Moderate abnormal	20	1
Slight abnormal		3
Borderline		7
Normal		1
Total	25	12

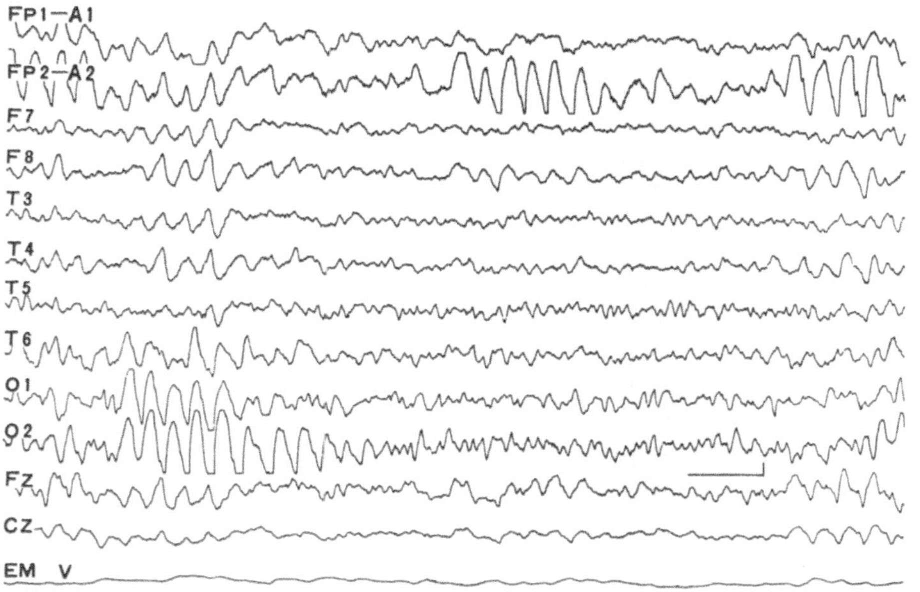

Fig. 62. Posterior slow waves (P-slow) in the EEG of a 9-year-old male case. Such slow waves are seen within 1 or 2 years from onset of symptoms

usually between 2.5 and 4 Hz and monorhythmic high-voltage slow waves are found predominantly over the affected hemisphere.

Such EEG activity has been found in 19 of our 34 cases (56 %). Most patients manifest such activity within 1 or 2 years after onset of symptoms and it is noteworthy that all 12 of our juvenile cases in which EEG examination was undertaken within 1 year after onset showed such slow-wave activity.

Based on the fact that opening of the eyes or sleep results in a decrease or disappearance of the p-slow waves, it is thought that these waves have their origin in the brain stem. In general, high-voltage slow waves in the occipital region are not unusual in children and arise even in healthy children [3], as well as subsequent

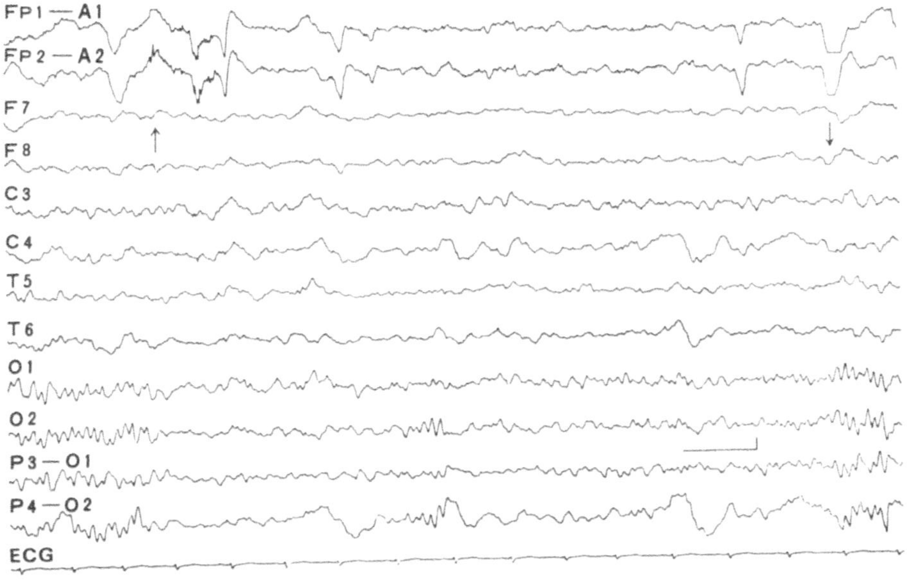

Fig. 63. Centrotemporal slow waves (CTslow) in the EEG of an 8-year-old female case. This activity is found most commonly more than 1 year from onset. ↑ eyes open, ↓ eyes closed

to head injury, epilepsy, or cerebrovascular disease. However, the fact that the p-slow waves are found predominantly on the affected side indicates that they have pathological significance.

5.2.1.2 Centrotemporal Slow Waves (CT Slow Waves)

CTslow waves are continuous polyrhythmic waves of mid to high voltage seen over the centrotemporal area of the affected hemisphere (Fig. 63). This activity is found most commonly more than 1 year after onset, and has been found in 10 of our 34 cases (29%). The fact that the wave form of the CTslow wave is unchanged by eye opening or sleep is thought to reflect a disturbance at the cortical level of the temporoparietal lobe. As compared with findings on the p-slow wave and the re-buildup phenomenon, those on the CTslow wave are not such specific findings.

5.2.1.3 Diffuse Slow Waves

Diffuse slow waves consist primarily of relatively low voltage theta waves and are seen many years after the onset of symptoms of moyamoya disease (Fig. 64). Eye opening does not readily suppress the diffuse slow waves and they are consequently thought to be indicative of a nonspecific chronic state of inhibition of electrical activity of the brain. In all of our cases, those who demonstrated diffuse slow wave activity also showed signs of mental retardation.

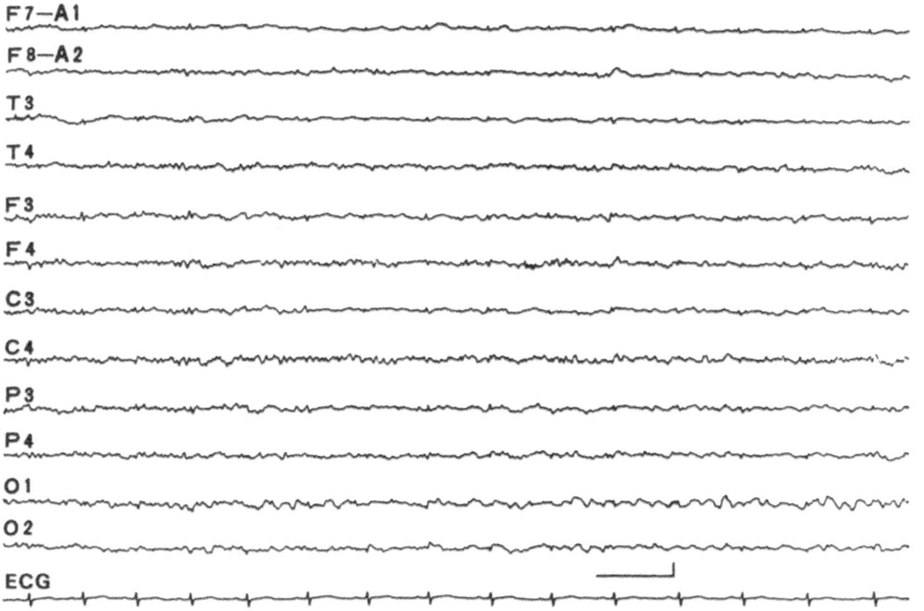

Fig. 64. Diffuse slow waves in the EEG of a 13-year-old male case. This activity is seen many years after onset

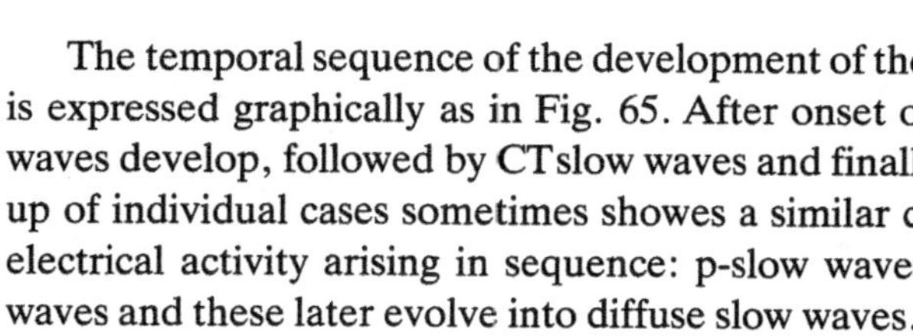

Fig. 65. Correlation between intervals from onset to EEG examination and the types of slow waves in 34 juvenile cases

The temporal sequence of the development of these three types of EEG waves is expressed graphically as in Fig. 65. After onset of moyamoya disease, p-slow waves develop, followed by CTslow waves and finally diffuse slow waves. Follow-up of individual cases sometimes showes a similar course with all three kinds of electrical activity arising in sequence: p-slow waves gradually become CT slow waves and these later evolve into diffuse slow waves.

There have also been reports of cases [340] in which frequent TIA-like attacks have disappeared simultaneously with the disappearance of p-slow waves and the emergence of CT slow waves. As TIA-like attacks reappeared, p-slow waves reappeared and as the symptoms became less severe, again the CT slow waves returned.

We believe that among these varieties of slow-wave activity p-slow waves are unique to moyamoya disease. That is, in moyamoya disease, disturbances of the area perfused by the middle cerebral artery are most severe and, since the circulation within the posterior cerebral artery is normally well maintained, centrencephalic monorhythmic slow waves most easily arise in the occipital region. Abnormal activity is next seen over the frontal lobe, where disturbances are mild. As the moyamoya disease progresses, these p-slow waves become nonspecific EEG abnormalities, such as the CTslow waves and eventually diffuse slow waves.

5.2.2 Electroencephalic Changes During Hyperventilation

The appearance of abnormal EEGs induced by hyperventilation is the most characteristic finding in juvenile moyamoya disease. Yoshii and Kudo [354, 355] first reported that diffuse slow waves are induced by hyperventilation in such juvenile cases and they argued that the cause for this was a decrease in $PaCO_2$ due to hyperventilation and a consequent decrease in cerebral blood flow which leads to brain hypoxia.

Yamamoto et al. [348] also observed a marked buildup due to hyperventilation and prolongation of slow waves following such hyperventilation. They noted, however, that the site of origin of such prolonged slow waves does not necessarily agree with the site at which clinical symptoms indicate a lesion exists. We have previously noted that in juvenile moyamoya disease after the buildup has subsided or a basic rhythm has appeared following hyperventilation, some 20–50 s later there is marked reappearance of the slow waves. This phenomenon has been labeled »re-buildup« [9, 135] (Fig. 66).

Even in cases in which there is no decrease in the slow-wave activity following hyperventilation, but rather further increases in slow-wave activity, the slow waves arising after hyperventilation are found to be more irregular in nature and of low frequency [278, 308], — in sharp contrast to the strong monorhythmic slow waves seen during hyperventilation. Such irregular and low-frequency waves are thought to be fundamentally similar to the re-buildup phenomenon (Fig. 67).

Re-buildup generally disappears within 10 min, but there are occasionally cases where it will last for ½ h. During the appearance of re-buildup, a child will sometimes feel at the point of losing consciousness, and there are also cases of TIA-like attacks. Re-buildup is usually found within several years of onset of moyamoya disease [269]. Among our 28 cases in which the effects of hyperventilation were tested, 23 (81%) showed re-buildup and among the 30 such cases of Karasawa et al. [112], 24 (80%) showed re-buildup.

As mentioned above, the fact that the buildup phenomenon consists of high-voltage monorhythmic slow waves suggests that these waves are of deep (brain stem) origin. In contrast, although the re-buildup phenomenon is also high voltage, it consists of more irregular and lower frequency components, suggesting that it may be of cortical or subcortical origin.

Moreover, in juvenile moyamoya cases in which the re-buildup has been identified, measurements of transcutaneous PO_2 and PCO_2 over the skin of the

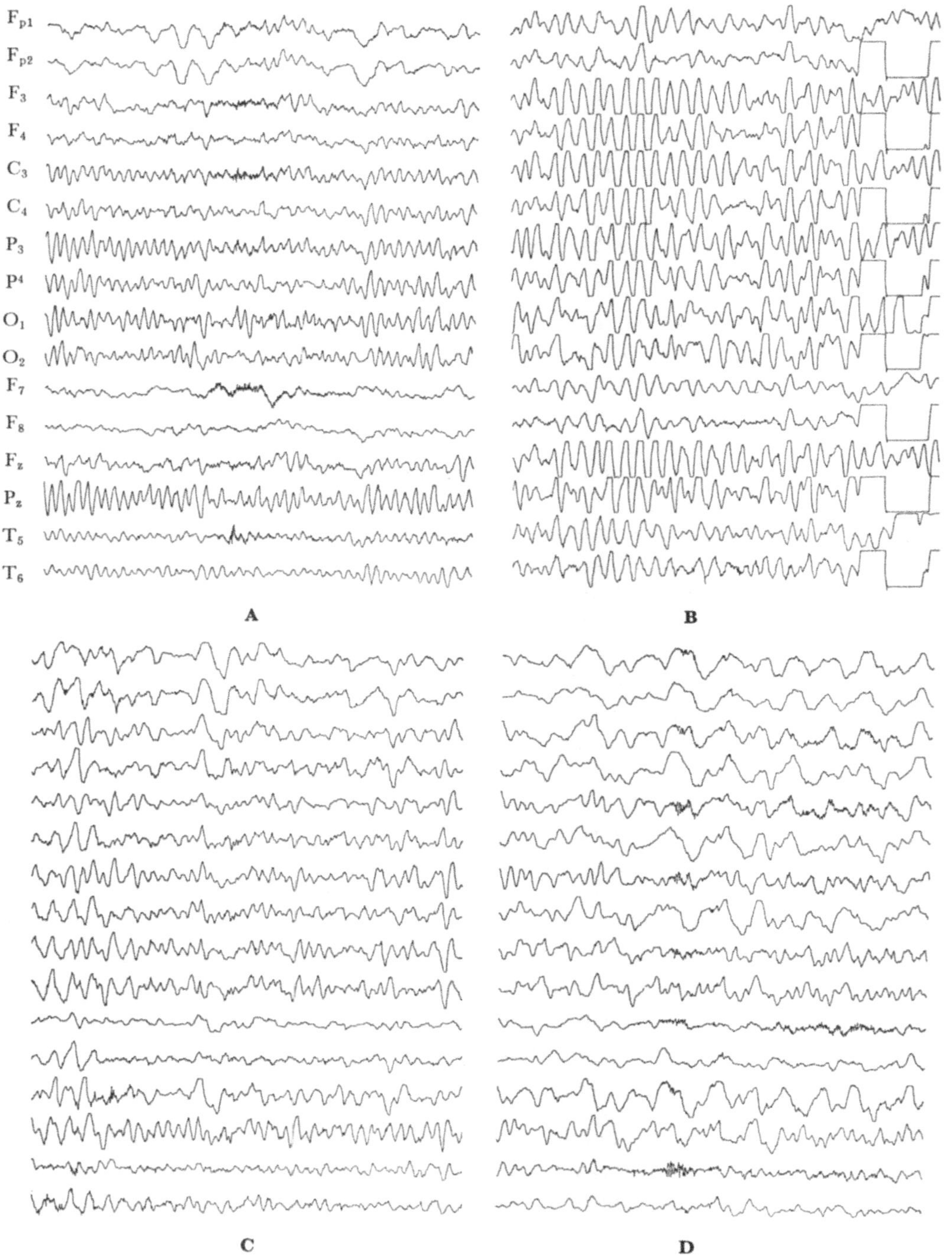

Fig. 66 A–D. A 6-year-old male case. **A** At rest; **B** during hyperventilation (buildup); **C** 30 s after hyperventilation (reappearance of basic pattern); **D** 60 s after hyperventilation (re-buildup)

A

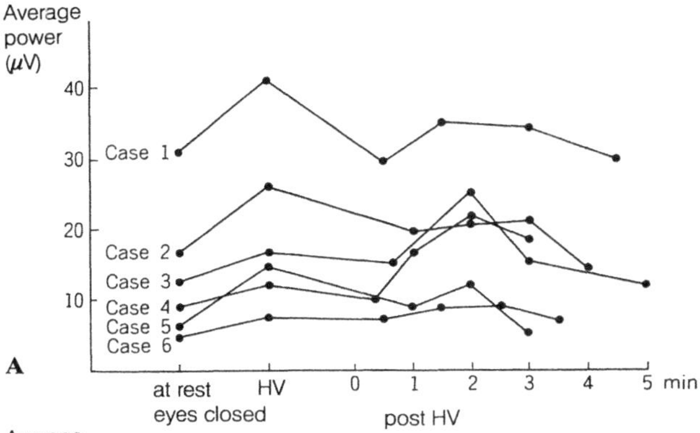

B

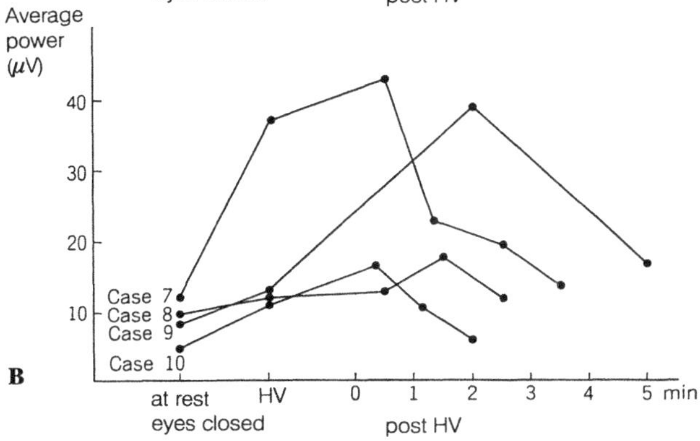

Fig. 67 A, B. Sequential changes in average power of δ-waves at the most intensely detected region, and hyperventilation (*HV*). **A** In cases 1–6, δ-waves decreased once after the cessation of hyperventilation; however they reappeared thereafter. **B** In cases 7–10, further increase in slow waves following hyperventilation was observed. However, the slow waves arising after hyperventilation were found to be more irregular in nature and of low frequency, whereas the monorhythmic slow waves were seen during hyperventilation

anterior thorax, which show good correlation with PaO_2 and $PaCO_2$, showed a gradual decrease in PCO_2 due to hyperventilation, which recovered gradually 30–50 s following the termination of the hyperventilation. In contrast, during hyperventilation and for 20–30 s following hyperventilation, tissue PO_2 remained at a high level, after which a sharp fall was seen due to the decrease in the rate of respiration where tissue PO_2 fell to 50–60 mmHg. Several minutes were then required for recovery of the PO_2 from this low level. In other words, while the buildup phenomenon appears during a fall in PCO_2 and when there is a high level of PO_2, the re-buildup phenomenon appears during the recovery of PCO_2 while it is still at a low level and PO_2 is at a markedly low level (Fig. 68). Measurement of PO_2 and PCO_2 during expiration showed a similar trend. Moreover, in those cases in which buildup and re-buildup were seen during and after hyperventilation of room air, hyperventilation of 8% CO_2 and 92% O_2 resulted in an extremely mild

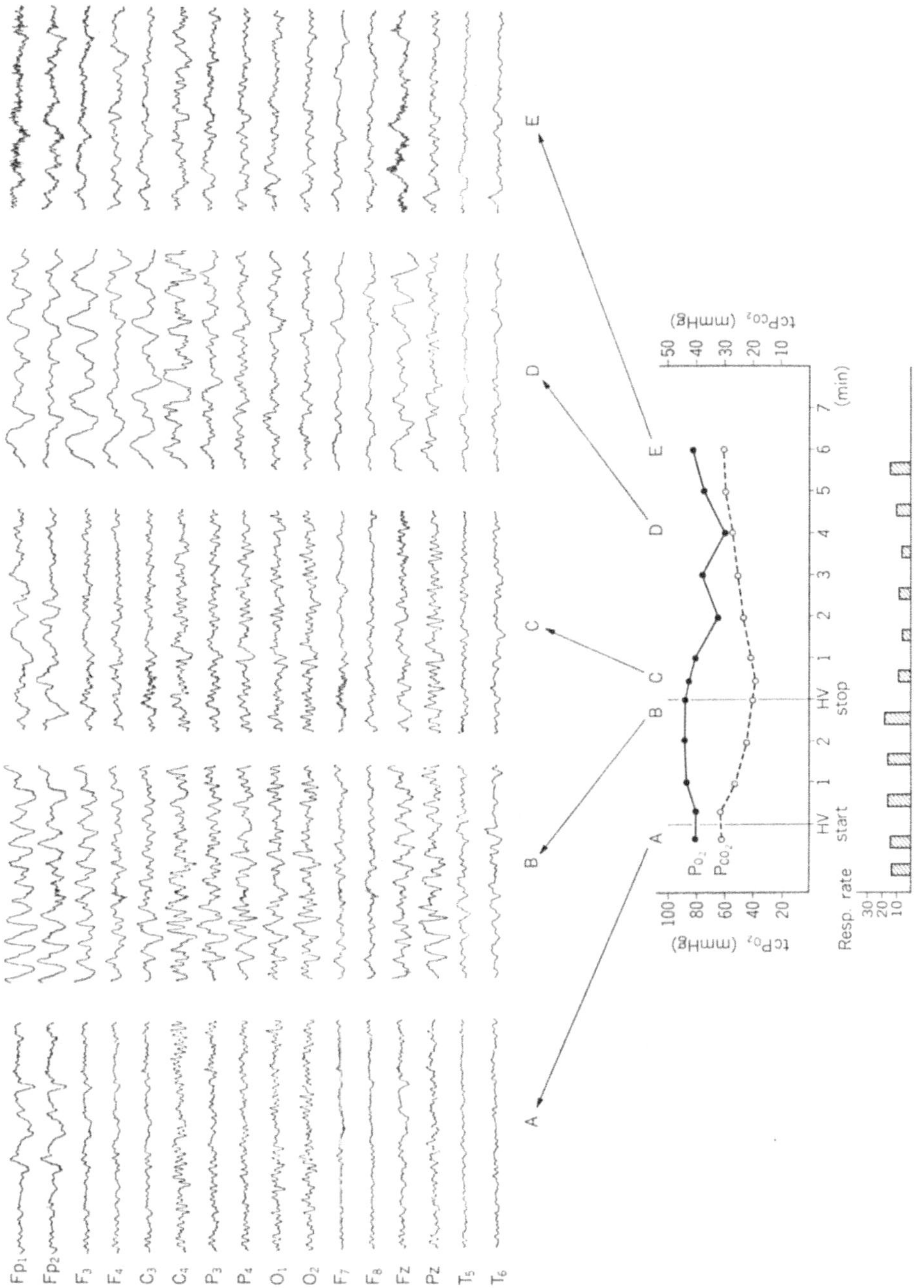

Fig. 68. Changes in EEG findings, transcutaneous PO_2 and PCO_2 over the skin of the anterior thorax and respiratory rates by hyperventilation

or no buildup or re-buildup at all. Hyperventilation with 100% O_2 then resulted in a marked buildup, but only slight or no re-buildup.

From the above findings, it is thought that buildup is associated with decreases in PCO_2 and re-buildup is associated with decreases in both PCO_2 and PO_2. With regard to the wave forms, it was found that a decrease in PCO_2 during hyperventilation had effects on the brain stem, resulting in the appearance of monorhythmic buildup. In contrast, a decrease in PO_2 following cessation of hyperventilation had effects at a cortical or subcortical level, resulting in the appearance of a polyrhythmic re-buildup.

5.2.3 Epileptic Discharge

Children with moyamoya disease often experience TIA-like attacks which can easily be mistaken for epileptic attacks, but convulsions are found in only 16% of juvenile moyamoya cases [207]. Spike or sharp waves are seen in the EEG in 12%–17% [74, 111, 207] and the wave forms are typically irregular spikes and waves, sharp waves over the temporal lobe, frontal small spikes, or 6- and 14-Hz positive spikes [88].

Kamio et al. [97] noted 6- and 14-Hz positive spikes in 5 of their 12 juvenile cases of moyamoya disease and we have seen similar spikes in 3 of our 34 cases. Gibbs et al. [50] have argued that such positive spikes are conducted to the cortex from the thalamus or hypothalamus. These positive spikes present an interesting problem with regard to the essential nature of moyamoya disease, but the clinical significance of these waves remains unclear.

5.3 Electroencephalography in Adult Cases of Moyamoya Disease

In comparison with the EEG findings in juvenile cases of moyamoya disease, those in adult cases have relatively few noteworthy characteristics (Table 8) [180]. Abnormalities in the EEG are mild, but there is often a decrease in the background activity either bilaterally or unilaterally, i.e., a decrease in the frequency of the basic rhythm, slow waves, or lazy activity over the affected hemisphere. Although there are often cortical irregular slow waves, corresponding to CTslow waves, there is nothing in the adult EEG comparable to the characteristic p-slow waves in juvenile cases. It is rare that re-buildup is seen. Among the 18 adult cases which we have tested during hyperventilation, only 1 showed re-buildup [269].

5.4 Evoked Potentials

Thus far, there have been only a very few published reports concerning evoked potentials in moyamoya disease. Honma et al. [79] have reported that in cases with neurological deficits due to cerebral infarction, abnormalities of somatosensory evoked potentials are seen on the side of the lesion, whereas in cases of TIA alone, there are no abnormalities of these evoked potentials. Tsuchimoto et al. [333] have reported that in juvenile cases of frequent TIA-like attacks, hyperventilation results in a low-amplitude N-55 component, and they have pointed out the similarities of the EEGs of such patients with re-buildup findings. There are also reports of a normal auditory brain stem response [79] in moyamoya disease, supporting the idea that moyamoya disease is a lesion located supratentorially.

5.5 Summary

The background electrical activity and evoked potentials recorded in cases of moyamoya disease are discussed, with particular emphasis on unusual EEG findings in juvenile cases. The sequence of EEG changes seen during and subsequent to hyperventilation are unique to juvenile moyamoya disease. Henceforth, further analysis of the EEG findings with control of various parameters would be of extreme value for delineating the essential nature of moyamoya disease.

6 Computerized Tomography

6.1 Introduction

Cerebral angiography is essential for the diagnosis of moyamoya disease and much research has been done on the nature of this disease based upon the findings obtained by means of angiography. It is, however, difficult to understand the nature of the morphological changes in brain tissue which are involved in the neurological changes in brain tissue which are involved in the neurological deficits and functional prognosis of moyamoya disease solely based upon cerebral angiography.

In recent years, computerized tomography has gained rapid acceptance as a diagnostic technique which cannot be overlooked in the diagnosis and treatment of lesions due to cerebral infarction or intracerebral hemorrhage. Consequently, computerized tomography has also proven effective in moyamoya disease, which produces symptoms due to brain ischemia or brain hemorrhage. Moreover, the fact that it is a noninvasive technique is also of particular importance for studying juvenile moyamoya cases. In this chapter, the use of computerized tomography in the diagnosis of moyamoya disease is discussed.

6.2 Unenhanced Scan

Abnormal findings obtained by computerized tomography include the following four types in moyamoya disease: low-density areas, cortical atrophy, ventricular dilatation, and high-density areas. The first three findings are due primarily to cerebral ischemia [40, 63, 64, 110, 177, 179, 297, 329, 358], whereas the high-density areas are known to indicate intracerebral hemorrhage [7, 12, 200, 301, 302].

The low-density areas in moyamoya disease are characteristically bilateral and occur as multiple lesions (Fig. 69). It is unusual for the lesion in moyamoya disease to coincide with the perfusion area of only one of the trunk arteries of the brain, as is commonly found in brain infarction due to the occlusion of one of these arteries. The site of appearance is both cortical and subcortical and is frequently found over the frontal, parietal, and temporal lobes. In contrast, the cerebral basal ganglia where moyamoya vessels are present often are normodensity and low-density areas not found in the cerebellum or brain stem.

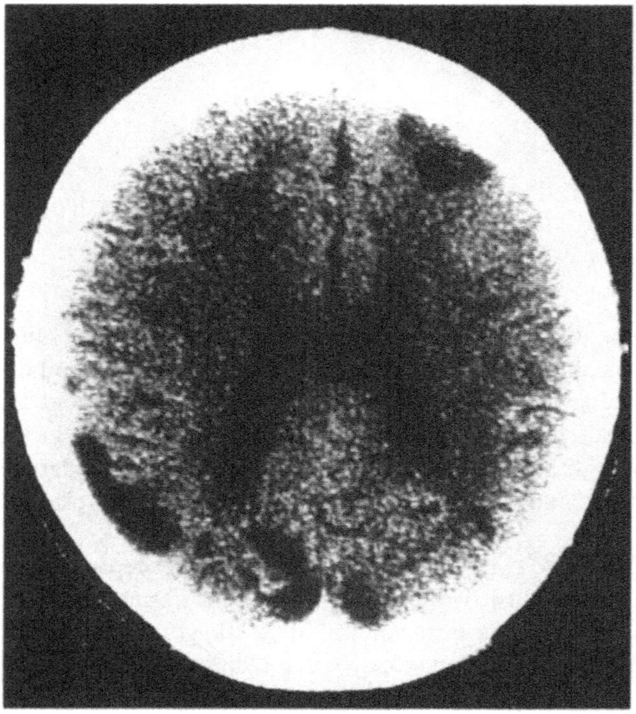

Fig. 69. A 6-year-old male case. Multiple low-density areas were seen bilaterally

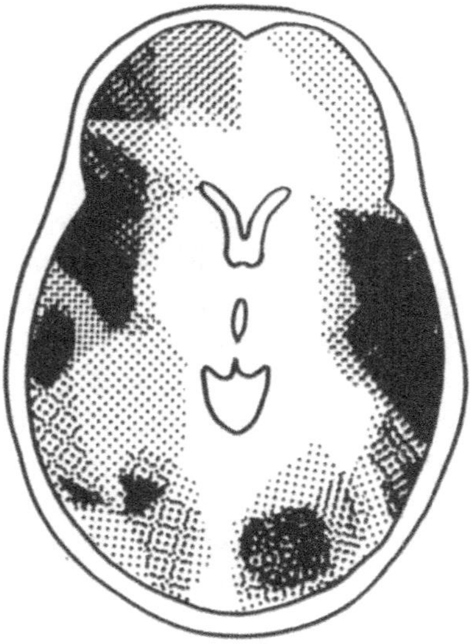

Fig. 70. The sites and extents of low-density areas in juveniles (ten cases)

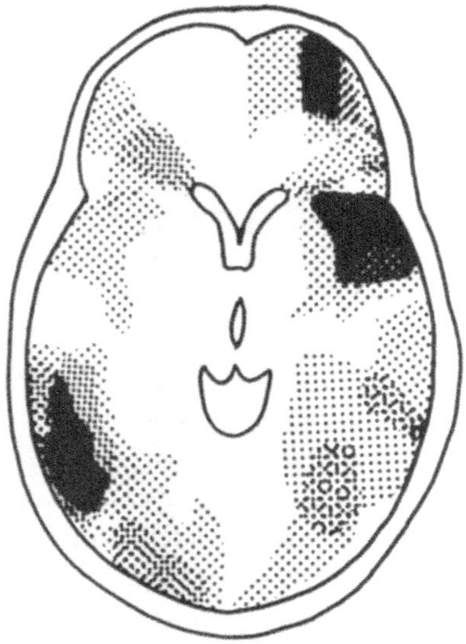

Fig. 71. The sites and extents of low-density areas in adults (ten cases)

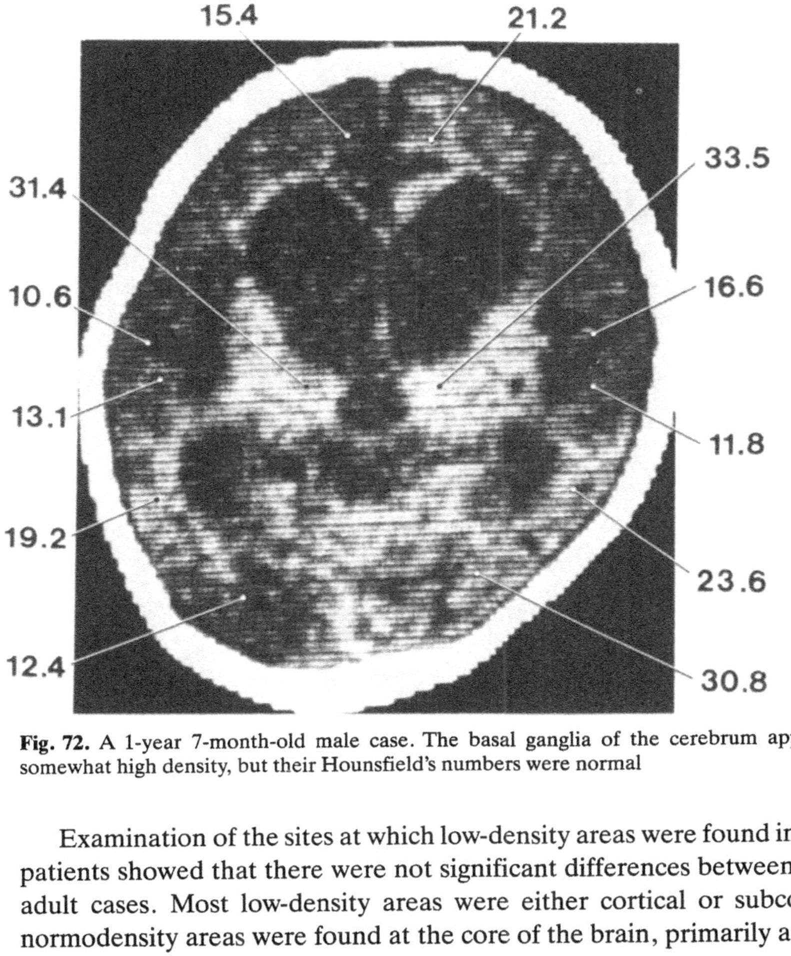

Fig. 72. A 1-year 7-month-old male case. The basal ganglia of the cerebrum appeared to be of somewhat high density, but their Hounsfield's numbers were normal

Examination of the sites at which low-density areas were found in our series of patients showed that there were not significant differences between juvenile and adult cases. Most low-density areas were either cortical or subcortical, while normodensity areas were found at the core of the brain, primarily at the cerebral basal ganglia (Figs. 70,71) [297].

It should be noted that regions of the basal ganglia normally appear visually to be of somewhat high density, but due to the low density of surrounding brain tissue the absorption values of this region were not high in any of the cases studied in our series (Fig. 72).

Cerebral atrophy in moyamoya disease is generally bilateral and can be seen as the widening of cerebral sulci, primarily in the frontal lobe, widening of the sylvian fissure and widening of the interhemispheric fissure (Fig. 73). Ventricular dilatation is sometimes seen of the lateral ventricles bilaterally and of the third ventricle; however, this ventricular dilatation is thought not to be due to internal hydrocephalus, but to cerebral atrophy (Fig. 72). It should also be noted that the degree of ventricular dilatation, the degree of cerebral atrophy, and the degree and extent of such low-density areas are known to correlate with the development of neurological symptoms and with mental deterioration.

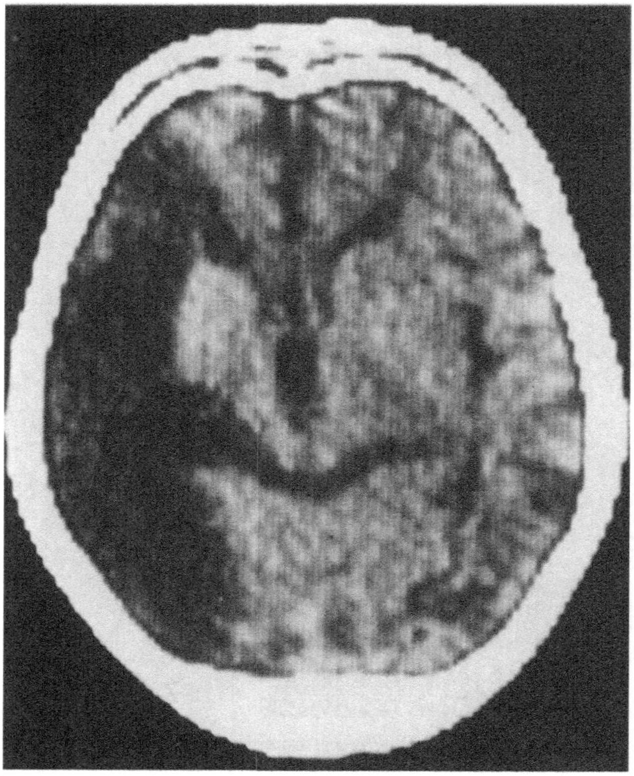

Fig. 73. A 10-year 10-month-old female case. Enlargements of sulci and interhemispheric fissure, etc. due to cerebral atrophy were seen

Next, with regard to the high-density areas observed in moyamoya disease, it is of course well known that high-density areas indicate intracranial hemorrhage. However, as described in the chapter on symptomatology, although the onset of symptoms is due to hemorrhage in most adult cases, the source of the hemorrhage is not, as was previously thought, an abnormally weakened vessel which ruptures into the subarachnoid space at the base of the brain. Rather, since the introduction of computerized tomography, it has become known that subarachnoid hemorrhage in moyamoya disease is infrequent, and paraventricular intracerebral hematoma together with ventricular rupture is most common (Fig. 74).

Computerized tomography data from 222 cases [208] of moyamoya disease have been collected by Professor Fumio Gotoh of the Research Committee on Spontaneous Occlusion of the Circle of Willis of the Ministry of Health and Welfare, Japan. According to those statistics, low-density areas are seen subcortically in 36%, cortically in 28%, and at the basal ganglia in 6% (Table 9). High-density areas are seen at the basal ganglia in 11%, subcortically in 10%, and intraventricularly in 5% (Table 10). It is thought that there are changes with time

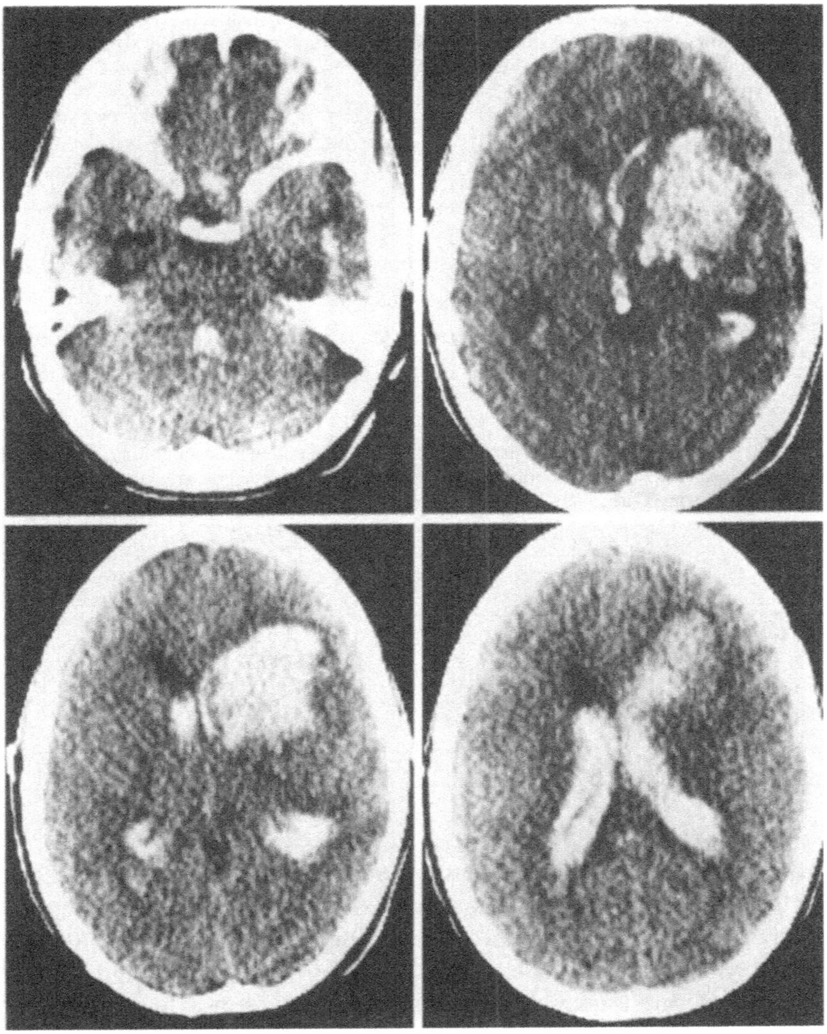

Fig. 74. A 56-year-old female case. Rupturing of intracerebral hematoma to the ventricle

in the density of brain tissue in moyamoya disease, but unfortunately, in the available statistics, there is no mention of the period from onset until examination.

6.3 Enhanced Scan

Moyamoya disease in both children and adults involves deficits in cerebral circulation due to brain ischemia. Consequently, when contrast medium is used and the sequential changes are followed from the time of onset, it is easy to

Table 9. Sites and frequencies of low-density areas on CT scan classified by clinical types of attack. The site of appearance of low-density areas is mainly both cortical and subcortical, and they rarely appear in cerebral basal ganglia. Moreover, the frequency of appearance of low-density areas is naturally high in ischemic types (Nishimoto and Oube [208])

Types of attack	Sites			
	No low-density area (%)	Cortex (%)	Subcortex (%)	Basal ganglia (%)
Hemorrhage (*n* = 9)	52	10	29	10
Convulsion (*n* = 21)	52	24	33	5
Completed stroke (*n* = 64)	8	52	59	5
Transient ischemic attack (*n* = 46)	57	35	26	2
Total (*n* = 222)	40	28	36	6

Table 10. Sites and frequencies of high-density areas classified by clinical types of attack. The site of appearance of high-density areas is characteristically seen at the paraventricular area in subcortex and basal ganglia (Nishimoto and Oube [208])

Types of attack	Sites				
	No low-density area (%)	Cortex (%)	Subcortex (%)	Basal ganglia (%)	Intraventricle (%)
Hemorrhage (*n* = 91)	43	3	20	24	13
Convulsion (*n* = 21)	90	0	5	5	0
Completed stroke (*n* = 64)	80	0	5	2	0
Transient ischemic attack (*n* = 46)	93	2	2	2	0
Total (*n* = 222)	71	2	10	11	5

imagine that within the areas of low density, such as commonly seen in cases of brain infarction, there might be cases showing contrast enhancement effects. In fact, however, such enhancement is rare. The reason for this fact is that, although onset begins as symptoms of brain ischemia, the symptoms disappear quickly and such TIA-like attacks are repeated, leading to a gradual increase in the extent of the low-density areas. The resultant brain ischemia is consequently different from that due to the sudden occlusion of trunk arteries of the brain and this is thought to be the reason why so few moyamoya cases show enhancement effects. Particularly among infant cases, it is also true that examination using contrast medium is not often performed in the early period following onset.

In the following section, a case experienced at our clinic will be outlined in which enhancement effects were found.

Case Study: 6-year 7-month-old Girl. From July of 1980 (age 5 1/2 years), the patient experienced frontal headaches three or four times monthly, occasionally accompanied by nausea and vomiting. On 21 May 1981, she complained of a headache in the morning. At about 3 p.m. while climbing the stairs, she suddenly

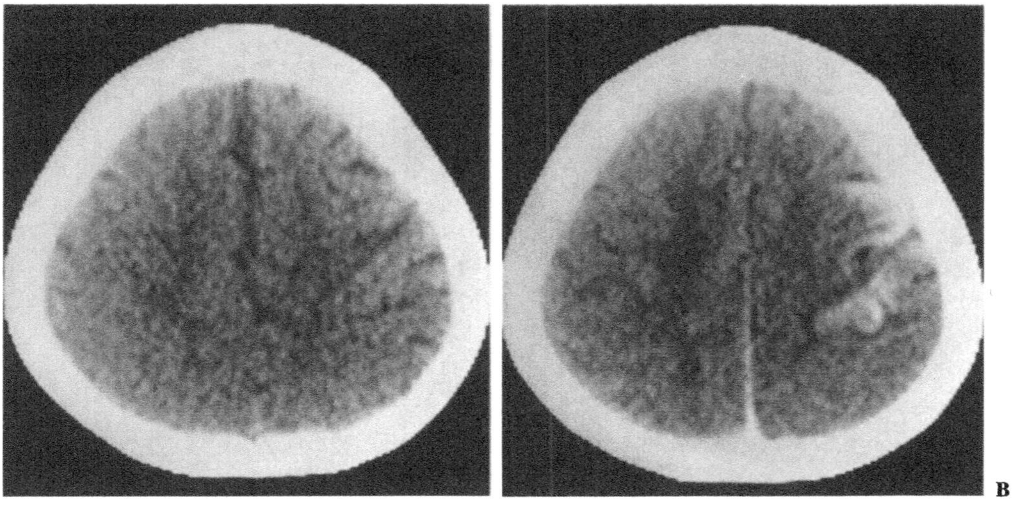

Fig. 75 A, B. A 6-year 7-month-old female case. A Unenhanced CT taken 6 days after the appearance of mild paresis of the left upper extremity showed a slight low-density area confined to the sulci of the right parietal lobe. B These low-density areas with surrounding brain tissue were enhanced by contrast medium (B)

fell due to left hemiparesis. The paresis disappeared completely in about 20 s, but she was admitted to a local clinic for further examination on the following day. Cerebral angiograms resulted in a diagnosis of moyamoya disease. On 13 July she experienced mild analgesia of the left upper extremity which did not improve with time. On 17 July she was admitted to our clinic. On admission, consciousness was clear, but there was a loss of strength confined to the left upper extremity. Computerized tomography taken on 22 July showed slight low density confined to the sulci of the right parietal lobe (Fig. 75). Injection of contrast medium showed enhancement effects (Fig. 75), which gradually became more distinct. These effects were visible until an examination on 6 August.

One of the points of interest in the computerized tomography of moyamoya cases is the question of whether or not contrast enhancement effects can be seen in the region of the moyamoya vessels. According to various authors [63, 110, 358] enhancement effects occur in less than half of the cases and, contrary to the prediction based upon angiographical findings, moyamoya vessels at the base of the brain are not easily enhanced due to the injection of contrast medium.

With regard to the detection of such moyamoya vessels, Asari et al. [14] have made various studies of the concentration and timing of injection of the contrast medium in order that these vessels may become clearly delineated. They have carried out computerized tomography at the time when the iodine concentration of the arterial blood is high and report success in detecting the moyamoya vessels using the intravenous minimum-dose bolus injection method.

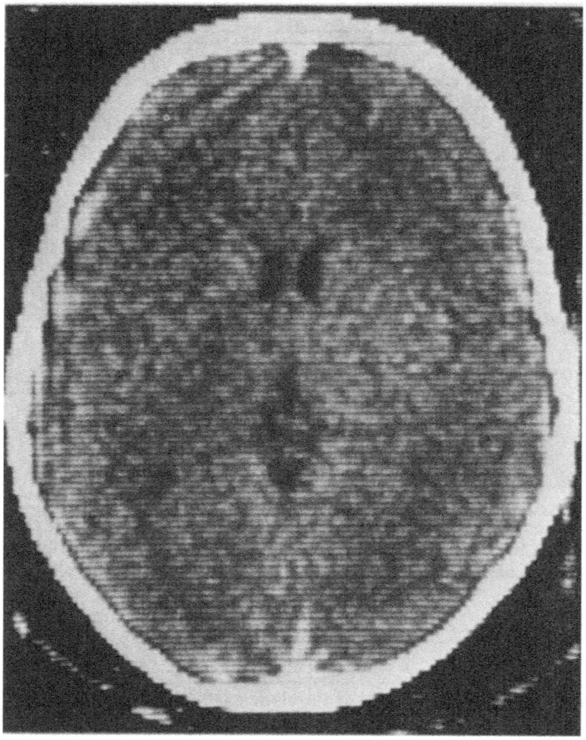

Fig. 76. A 10-year 5-month-old male case. Almost normal CT findings were observed in this case, even though the angiogram showed stage 5 of basal moyamoya

6.4 Stage of Moyamoya Disease and Computerized Tomography

In previous chapters, we have noted that moyamoya disease typically begins as stenosis of the carotid bifurcation and shows dynamic changes with time until the entire internal carotid arterial system is no longer visible angiographically. We have made a study of the correlation between the six stages of moyamoya vessels at the base of the brain, as seen angiographically, and the extent and degree of the low-density areas seen in computerized tomography. Contrary to a previous study [357], where a close correlation was found between angiographical and computerized tomographical findings, in the current series a clear correlation was not always found. Specifically, although most moyamoya cases which were at stage 4, 5 or 6 angiographically also showed manifest abnormalities in computerized tomography, there were, albeit infrequently, cases which showed stage-5 lesions in angiograms, but had almost normal computerized tomography (Fig. 76). This lack of agreement between the angiographical and computerized tomographical findings is thought to be due to the presence of cases in which, despite a decrease in blood flow through the internal carotid arterial system, there is retrograde flow through the normally preserved vertebrobasilar arterial system or there is blood supplied via collateral pathways, such as often found in ethmoidal or vault moyamoya. Consequently, cerebral infarction in such cases is not advanced.

6.5 Conclusion

The predominant abnormal findings in unenhanced scans were ventricular dilatation, brain atrophy, and low-density areas thought to be due to prolonged brain ischemia. Moreover, high-density areas due to intracranial hemorrhage were also common. It was found that the extent and degree of these findings were closely related to the severity of neurological symptoms. With regard to enhanced scans, contrast enhancement effects have been experienced only rarely, although this is thought to be due to the fact that enhanced scans have been obtained in the early period following onset in only a small number of cases. Moreover, enhancement of moyamoya vessels present at the basal ganglia has not been as marked as might be expected when using conventional methods for infusion of the contrast medium. Various combinations of the timing of the infusion and different concentrations of contrast medium have been reported to produce greater clarity of enhancement effects. We were not able to identify a clear relationship between computerized tomography findings and the stage of the moyamoya disease as determined angiographically.

It is apparent that computerized tomography is an effective means for determining the nature of the lesion in moyamoya cases, for making follow-up studies, for determining the efficacy of the treatment, and for determining the prognosis.

7 Positron Emission Computerized Tomography

7.1 Introduction

The emergence of positron emission computerized tomography has had a great impact not only on the clinical diagnosis, but also on the basic understanding, of brain functions. Only this sophisticated tool has made it possible to evaluate various physiological factors in man with quantifiable, three-dimensional images noninvasively.

In this chapter, our preliminary experiences with positron emission computerized tomography in two cases of moyamoya disease will be presented, especially for the purpose of clarifying the relationship between the mechanism of the re-buildup phenomenon on EEG (Chap. 5) and brain functions.

7.2 Cases

Case 1 was a 13-year-old male who suffered from paraventricular hemorrhage in February 1983. The angiographical stage was 5 in the right side and 3 in the left (Chap. 3). Positron emission computerized tomography was performed 7 months after the onset.

Case 2 was a 17-year-old male who had had frequent TIA attacks since he was 4 years old. Perivascular sympathectomy and superior cervical ganglionectomy (Chap. 9) were performed on both sides 7 years ago. The angiographical stage was 6 on both sides.

Regional cerebral blood flow (CBF) and the cerebral metabolic rate of oxygen ($CMRO_2$) were measured by positron emission computerized tomography (ECAT II) [39] with the continuous inhalation method of $C^{15}O_2$ and $^{15}O_2$ [241] respectively. The patients were asked to hyperventilate for 3 min and scannings were performed before and after hyperventilation at the same single plane parallel to the orbitomeatal line, which includes the basal ganglia.

Posthyperventilation 5-min scanning showed marked changes in both CBF and $CMRO_2$. In case 1, a decrease in CBF was observed in the right hemisphere, where the angiographical stage was more advanced, while $CMRO_2$ decreased much more than CBF in whole brain regions (Figs. 77,78). In case 2, where there was no difference in the angiographical stage between the hemispheres, marked and symmetrical decreases in both CBF and $CMRO_2$ were observed (Fig. 79). However, the decrease in $CMRO_2$ was also more than that of CBF (Fig. 80).

Simultaneous EEG recordings showed typical re-buildup in both cases during the posthyperventilation 5-min scanning. Also, sequential changes in PaO_2 and $PaCO_2$ showed characteristic findings. A gradual decrease in $PaCO_2$ due to hyperventilation was observed, but there was gradual recovery following the cessation of hyperventilation and it returned to the prehyperventilation level at the time of posthyperventilation 5-min scanning. In contrast, the high level of PaO_2 due to hyperventilation fell sharply following the termination of hyperventilation probably because of the decrease in the rate of respiration. Even though PaO_2 gradually recovered, it remained at a low level at the time of posthyperventilation 5-min scanning (Fig. 81).

From the above findings, it seems unlikely that only the hemodynamic change following hyperventilation is responsible for the emergence of re-buildup on EEG, since there was a dissociation between the decrease in CBF and $CMRO_2$ in both cases. Instead, on the basis of these multiple physiological observations, the mechanism of re-buildup might be explained as follows; cerebral vessel constriction is produced due to the decrease in $PaCO_2$ following hyperventilation (Chap. 3) and it first appears as a CBF decrease on positron emission computerized tomography. Then, in addition to this decreased CBF, a delayed decrease in PaO_2 following hyperventilation results in the decrease in $CMRO_2$ which causes cerebral dysfunction, and thus it appears as the re-buildup phenomenon on the EEG. In other words, re-buildup is the manifestation of not only the hypoxic, but also the ischemic, state seen characteristically in moyamoya disease.

Although further study must be carried out before any definite conclusion can be reached, positron emission computerized tomographic study of moyamoya disease seems to provide us with an important clue in elucidating this disease.

Fig. 77. Case 1: 13-year-old male. Decreased $CMRO_2$ (oxygen consumption) was observed at scanning 5 min posthyperventilation

Fig. 78. Case 1: Changes in CBF and $CMRO_2$ between prehyperventilation and 5 min posthyperventilation. CBF was decreased mainly in the right hemisphere where the angiographical stage was more advanced. In contrast, the decrease in $CMRO_2$ was much greater than that in CBF in the whole brain regions

77
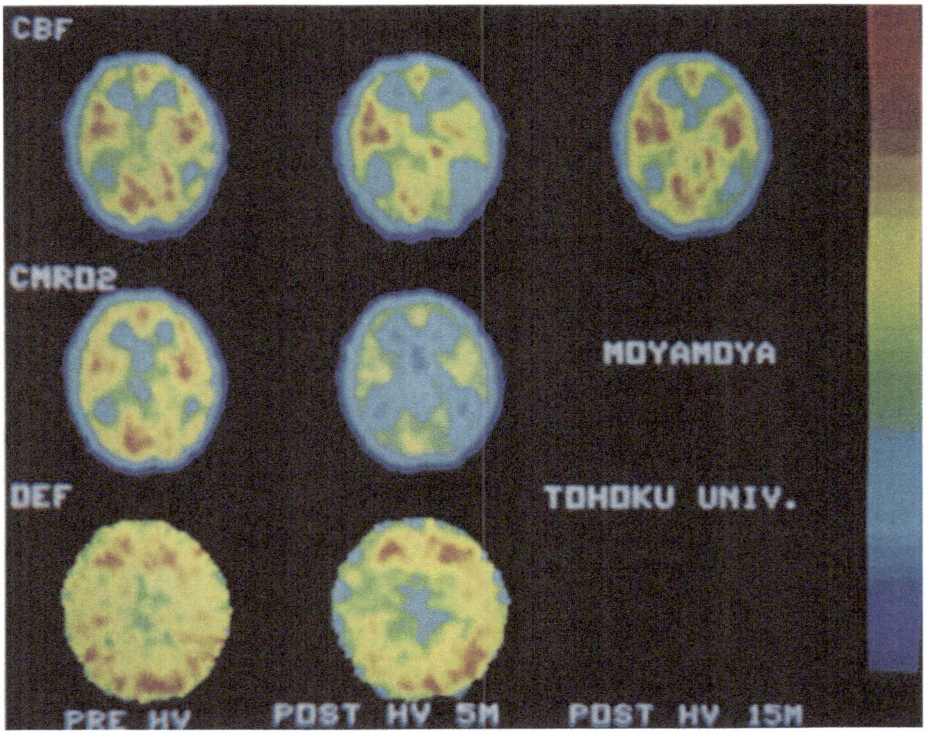
CBF
CMRO2
MOYAMOYA
DEF
TOHOKU UNIV.
PRE HV
POST HV 5M
POST HV 15M

78
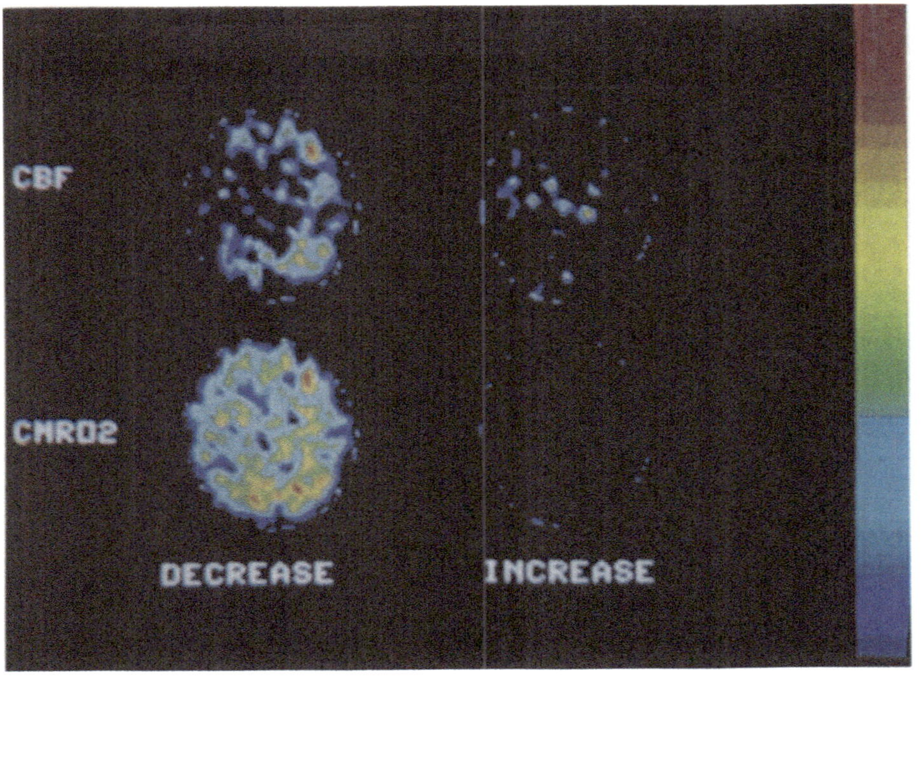
CBF
CMRO2
DECREASE
INCREASE

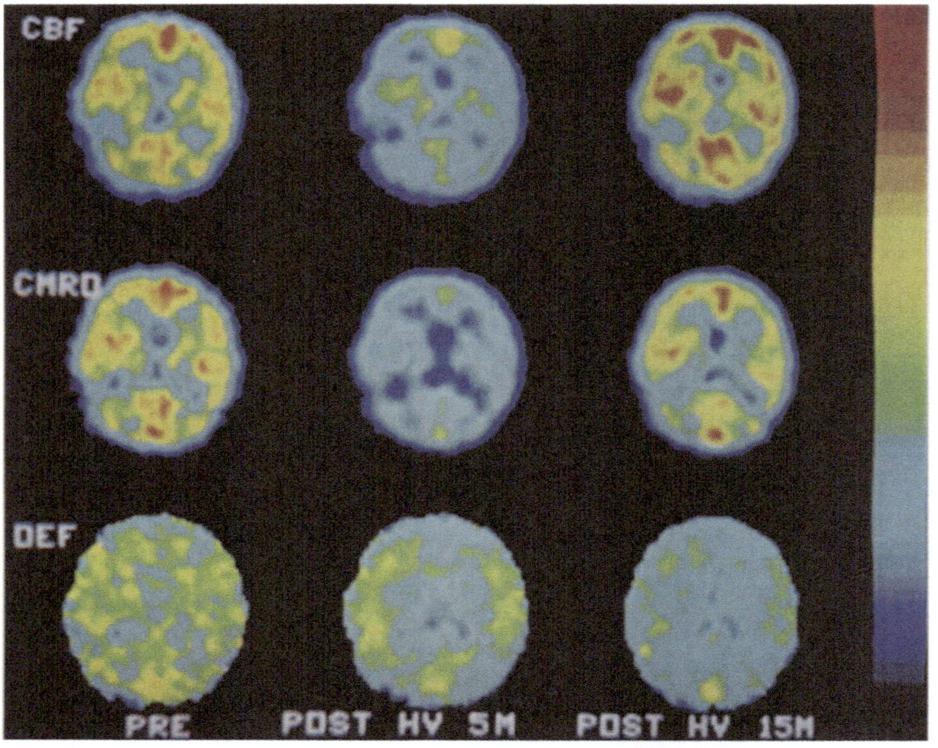
CBF
CMRO
OEF
PRE
POST HV 5M
POST HV 15M

79

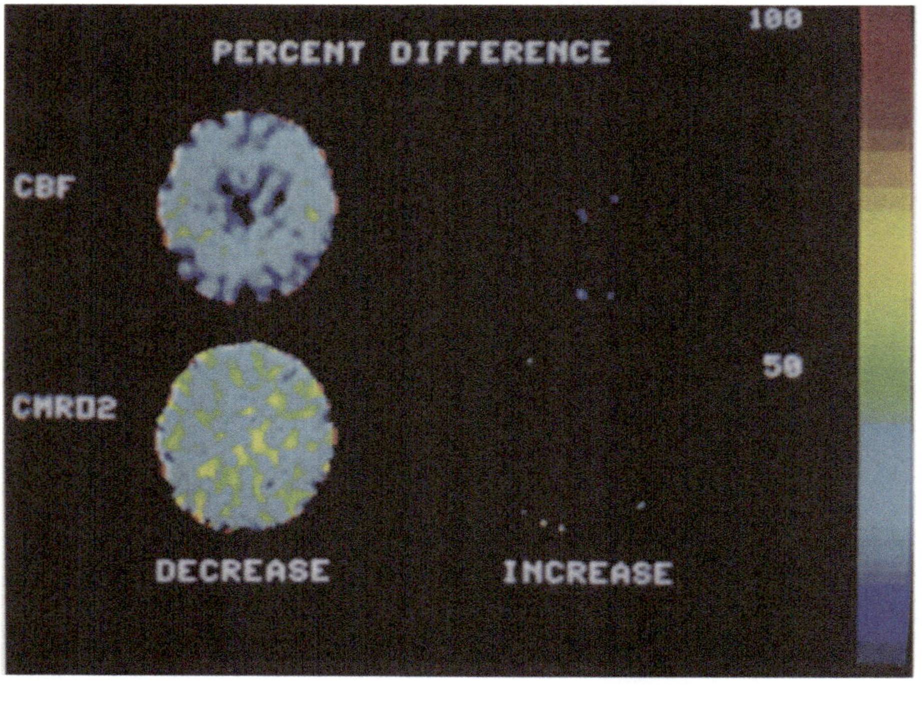
PERCENT DIFFERENCE
100
CBF
50
CMRO2
DECREASE
INCREASE

80

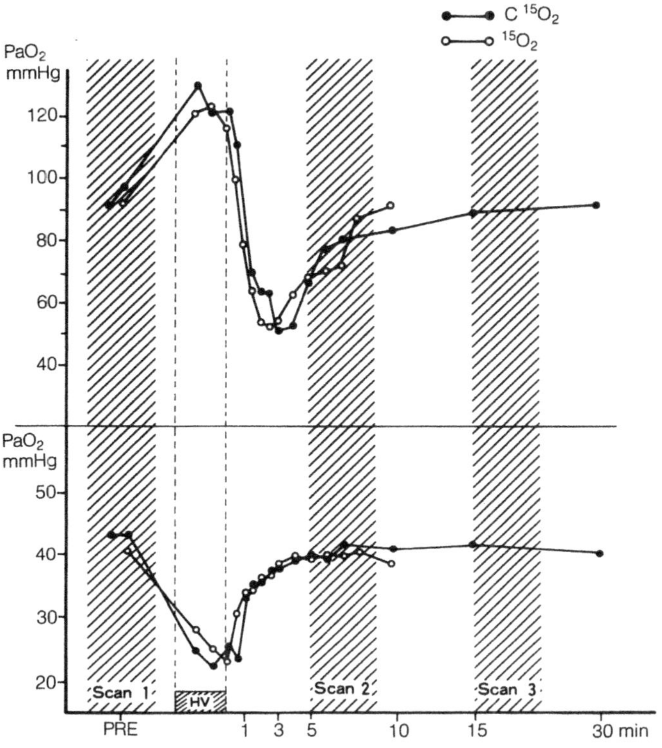

Fig. 81. Case 1: Sequential changes of PaO_2 and $PaCO_2$. At scanning 5 min posthyperventilation, $PaCO_2$ returned to its normal range; however, PaO_2 remained at a low level due to the decrease in the rate of respiration following hyperventilation

◄

Fig. 79. Case 2: 17-year-old male. Marked and symmetrical decrease in both CBF and $CMRO_2$ was observed at 5 min posthyperventilation, and they almost returned to prehyperventilation level at 15 min posthyperventilation

Fig. 80. Case 2: Percentage difference in CBF and $CMRO_2$ between prehyperventilation and 5 min posthyperventilation. Decrease in $CMRO_2$ was also more than that of CBF

8 Cerebral Hemodynamics

8.1 Introduction

The first report concerning the cerebral circulation in moyamoya disease was that byTakahashi et al. [303] in 1967, in which a classic nitrous oxide technique was used to study the average cerebral blood flow in six moyamoya cases. Several other studies using the same method have been reported since then [51, 52, 327, 328], and recently investigations using an argon inhalation method [113, 178] and radioisotope angiography [138, 166, 169, 221, 307] have also been reported. In addition, studies on regional cerebral blood flow (rCBF) using the ^{133}Xe intracarotid injection method have been numerous [69, 189, 190, 316] since the investigations of Uemura et al. [334] and Mizukawa [180] in 1975.

Unfortunately, in moyamoya disease there is considerable blood flow to the brain via pathways other than the internal carotid arterial system and this fact implies that measurement of the CBF of only the perfusion area of the internal carotid artery is not sufficient for a genuine understanding of the cerebral circulation of moyamoya disease.

In contrast to the above methods, the method for determining rCBF of moyamoya disease by means of ^{133}Xe intravenous injection, as reported by us in 1981 [224], requires minimal invasion, reflects the blood flow of all cerebral vessels, and also allows for rCBF measurements. Consequently, it is thought to be a superior means for determining CBF of this disease. Furthermore, recently developed methods for three-dimensional measurement of CBF using stable xenon-enhanced computerized tomography [53, 54, 55] and emission tomography are gradually making possible the determination of rCBF of deep portions of the brain and will undoubtedly contribute greatly to further elucidation of the cerebral circulation in moyamoya disease.

Finally, there has recently been considerable research on cerebral autoregulation following induced hypertension or hypotension and on the vascular reactivity to CO_2 inhalation and hyperventilation. Consequently, the vascular responsiveness in this lesion has gradually been elucidated.

In this chapter, the hemodynamics of moyamoya disease will be discussed on the basis of the reports of various authors. In addition, there will also be detailed discussion of the method for continuous measurement of CBF using ^{81m}Kr, developed by Ogawa et al. [223], with emphasis on the collateral circulation of the vertebrobasilar arterial system in moyamoya disease.

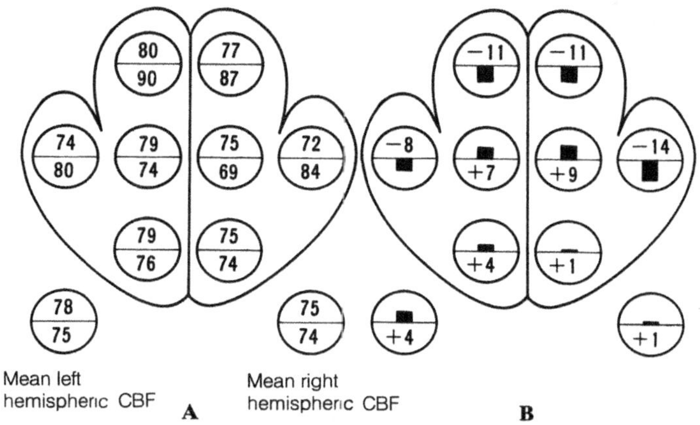

Fig. 82 A, B. rCBF of moyamoya disease in adult cases (^{133}Xe intravenous injection method). **A** rCBF in each brain region. *Upper values* show mean rCBF in four adult cases. *Lower values* show normal controls. **B** Percent age difference to normal subjects. The hemispheric CBF is virtually identical with normal subjects; however, there are low rCBF values in the frontal and temporal regions and relatively high rCBF in the parietal and occipital regions

8.2 Average Cerebral Blood Flow and Hemispherical Blood Flow

8.2.1 Cerebral Circulation in Adult Cases

Among investigations of the average CBF of the whole brain using the nitrous oxide method [51, 52, 303, 328, 329], most reports show that blood flow is within normal limits, providing that cases with neurological symptoms and those tested in the acute stage following onset are excluded. However, it has been observed that the severer the stenosis of the terminal portion of the internal carotid artery, the more marked is the decrease in cerebral blood flow and the oxygen consumption rate [33, 51, 52, 53, 54]. Similarly, using the ^{133}Xe intracarotid injection method [34, 180, 215, 334], hemispherical blood flow tends to parallel decreases in neurological symptoms. In asymptomatic cases or those with mild symptoms, however, nearly normal values for blood flow are said to be found.

Using the ^{133}Xe intravenous injection method, we have measured the hemispherical blood flow (CBF gray) in a group of adult cases (average age 24 years) in whom ischemic symptoms were found at the time of onset, but in whom ischemic symptoms had disappeared by the time of testing. The left and right hemispheres showed CBF values of 78 ± 4 and 75 ± 4 ml/min per 100 g brain, respectively, which were virtually identical with the mean of 75 ± 13 ml/min per 100 g found in a group of normal subjects (average age 30 years) [224] (Fig. 82).

In light of these data from our own and other laboratories, it can be said that the blood circulation of the whole brain or hemisphere in adult cases of moyamoya disease is within a normal range, with the exception of the acute period following onset and cases with severe neurological deficits.

8.2.2 Cerebral Circulation in Juvenile Cases

Karasawa et al. have reported a study of 17 juvenile cases of moyamoya disease with symptoms of cerebral ischemia, in whom the average CBF was measured using the argon method [113]. They found no difference in blood flow between cases with mild neurological deficits and those with severe ones, but they did find a decrease in the oxygen consumption rate and an increase in cerebrovascular resistance related to an increase in the severity of symptoms.

Nishimoto et al. [217] measured the hemispherical blood flow in five juvenile cases with no neurological deficits using the ^{133}Xe intracarotid injection method. They found no significant differences between those juvenile cases and the values obtained from normal adults. However, since it is known that the normal CBF in children is extremely high, a consideration of age factors in the above study suggests that the CBF in juvenile cases of moyamoya disease is below normal.

In our own study [224] using a ^{133}Xe intravenous injection method we have found the hemispherical blood flow of eight juvenile cases (ages ranging from 7 to 14 years, averaging 9.5) to be 82 ± 9 on the left and 83 ± 11 ml/min per 100 g on the right (Fig. 83). Although these values are higher than those in normal adults, again a consideration of the age of these patients suggests that there is a fall in CBF. That is, even in juvenile cases without marked neurological deficits, a comparison with the CBF values of normal children shows a decrease in cerebral circulation.

8.2.3 Regional Cerebral Blood Flow

In measurements using the ^{133}Xe intracarotid injection method [236, 334, 335], although there have been many cases showing an abnormal distribution of rCBF, there have been very few abnormalities of asymptomatic cerebral hemispheres.

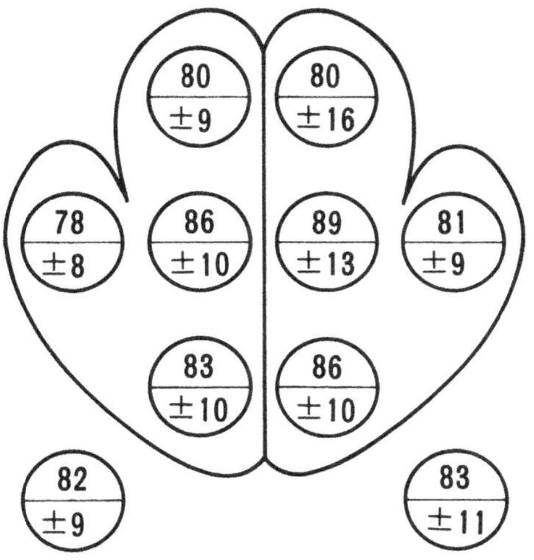

Fig. 83. rCBF of moyamoya disease in juvenile cases (^{133}Xe intravenous injection method). *Upper values* show mean rCBF of eight cases and *lower values* show standard deviation (SD). rCBF values are higher than those of normal adults; however, there are low rCBF values in the frontal and temporal lobes and relatively high rCBF values in the parietal and occipital lobes, the same as in the adult cases

Moreover, using the same method but measuring rCBF from the lateral aspect with a gamma camera [198] or an autofluoroscope [315, 335], or making a three-dimensional study with the stable xenon-enhanced CT[55], the rCBF values at the region containing moyamoya vessels have not shown high values in comparison with normal blood flow.

In our own study [224] using the ^{133}Xe intravenous injection method, the rCBF values obtained are thought to reflect not only the blood flow in the internal carotid arterial system, but also the flow through the vault moyamoya vessels via the external carotid arterial system and the flow through the vertebrobasilar arterial system. We found that in patients with no neurological symptoms there are low rCBF values in the frontal and temporal lobes and relatively high values in the parietal and occipital lobes as compared with normal CBF distribution in both juvenile and adult cases (Table 11, Figs. 82,83). These results are thought to indicate the importance in moyamoya diseases of blood circulation to the brain from the vertebrobasilar arterial system. Moreover, a comparison of these rCBF results with the six stages of basal moyamoya seen angiographically demonstrated that as the moyamoya lesion progressed the distribution of blood flow gradually changed from a predominance of flow to the frontal lobes to a predominance of flow to the parietal regions.

Table 11. Symptoms, EEG findings, and neuroradiological findings of rCBF-measured cases by the ^{133}Xe intravenous injection method

Case		Sex	Age (years)	Age (years) and symptom at onset		Symptom at examination	Re-buildup on EEG	CT findings	Angiographic stage	
									Left	Right
1	T.S.	M	7	6	TIA	(−)	(+++)		3	3
2	J.I.	M	7	6	TIA	(−)	(+)	Right frontal low	3	3
3	U.K.	F	7	4	TIA	(+)[a]	(+)	Ventricle dilatation	3	3
4	H.K.	F	8	6	TIA	(+)[a]	(+)	Ventricle dilatation	3	3
5	R.K.	F	9	4	TIA	(+)[b]	(−)	Right basal ganglia low	3	3
6	F.I.	F	11	4	TIA	(+)[b]	(+)	Left temporal low	4	4
7	U.G.	F	13	4	TIA	(−)	(+)		3	3
8	H.Y.	F	14	5	TIA	(−)	(+)		2	1
9	T.K.	M	18	7	TIA	(−)	(−)	Right frontal and left temporal low	2	2
10	T.S.	M	20	4	TIA	(+)[a]	(−)		4	3
11	T.Y.	M	33	20	TIA	(−)	(−)		4	4
12	M.S.	F	44	26	TIA	(+)[a]	(−)	Left temporal low	4	3

TIA, transient ischemic attack; re-buildup, refer to Chap. 5; angiographic stage, refer to Chap. 3

[a] Slight paresis [b] Slight mental retardation

Table 12. rCBF of moyamoya disease and normal control (ml/100 g brain per min) (Goto et al. [51–55]). In moyamoya disease, there is a slight decrease of blood flow in the frontal cortex and a slight increase in the occipital cortex

	Patients ($n = 5$)	Normal adults ($n = 5$)
Gray matter		
Frontal cortex	85.2+14.5	87.2+ 5.6
Occipital cortex	77.4+ 9.7	76.2+ 3.5
Putamen	85.9+10.2	91.5+ 7.2
Caudate nucleus	97.5+11.9	108.5+ 9.9
Thalamus	98.3+20.8	98.4+10.9
White matter		
Frontal deep portion	30.2+ 8.6	28.9+ 2.7
Occipital deep portion	31.1+ 4.8	26.1− 3.4

Using the stable xenon-enhanced CT technique for measuring rCBF, Gotoh et al. [55] also reported that there is a slight decrease of blood flow in the frontal cortex and a slight increase in the blood flow to the occipital cortex (Table 12).

From these various studies, it is evident that in moyamoya disease patients with neurological deficits there are marked abnormalities of the distribution of rCBF. In addition, it is thought that even in cases with few or no neurological symptoms whatsoever there is a tendency for there to be low rCBF values in the frontal and temporal regions and high values in the parietal and occipital regions, as compared with normal CBF distribution.

8.2.4 Differences in rCBF Values in the Perfusion Areas of the Internal Carotid Artery and the Vertebrobasilar Artery

A comparison of the perfusion areas of the internal carotid arterial system and the vertebrobasilar artery system was next made. The subjects of this study were three females and one male between the ages of 14 and 36 years. Two cases had TIA at onset, one had intraventricular hemorrhage, and moyamoya disease was discovered fortuitously in one case. In all four cases no neurological deficits were present at the time of testing and moyamoya disease was judged to be between stages 3 and 5 in all cases (Table 13).

Table 13. Cases of moyamoya disease in which a comparison of the perfusion areas of the internal carotid arterial system and vertebrobasilar arterial system was made

Case		Age and symptom at onset		Symptom at examination	Angiographic stage Left	Right	Side examined CBF
14Y	F	11Y	TIA	(−)	4	4	Left
28Y	F	27Y	TIA	(−)	3	3	Right
35Y	M	–		(−)	4	3	Left
36Y	F	36Y	IVH	(−)	4	5	Left

IVH, intraventricular hemorrhage

For measurement of cerebral blood flow, cannulation of the internal carotid artery or vertebrobasilar artery was done via the femoral artery and ^{81m}Kr was continuously infused through the catheter. Measurements were made of the internal carotid arterial system and the vertebrobasilar arterial system at 1-week intervals in each case.

In all of these patients, lateral aspects of the perfusion showed that there was not perfusion of the whole brain via the internal carotid arterial system, but rather only perfusion of the anterior half of the hemispheres. Moreover, cerebral circulation over the perfusion area was not homogeneous, but rather showed patches of more abundant and less abundant blood flow (Fig. 84). In contrast, perfusion through the vertebrobasilar arterial system showed blood flow not only to the cerebellum, but also to the posterior portion of the cerebral hemispheres and, in some cases, also perfusion of the temporal lobe and the posterior portion of the frontal lobe (Fig. 84). Moreover, the nonhomogeneous distribution of blood flow through the internal carotid artery is thought to be due to the perfusion from the external carotid arterial system through the vault moyamoya.

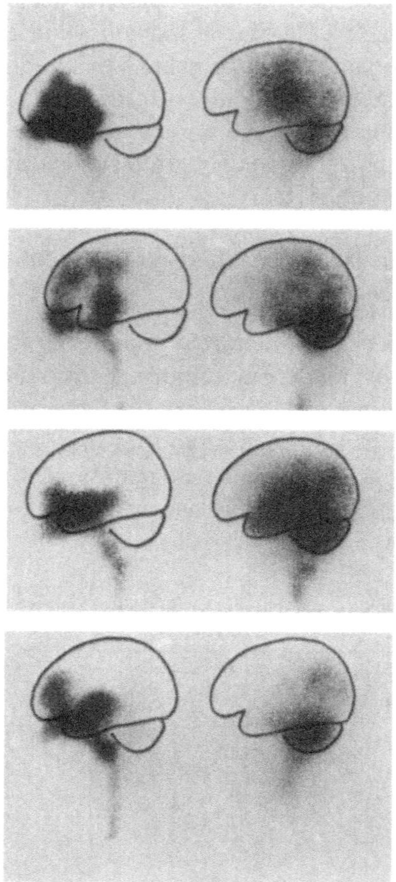

Fig. 84. Comparison of the perfusion areas of the internal carotid arterial system (*left*) and the vertebrobasilar arterial system (*right*). There is only perfusion of the anterior half of the cerebral hemispheres via the internal carotid arterial system; moreover, the cerebral circulation over the perfusion area is not homogeneous. In contrast, perfusion through the vertebrobasilar arterial system showed blood flow not only to the cerebellum but also to the posterior portion of the cerebral hemispheres and, in some cases, also perfusion of the temporal lobe and the posterior portion of the frontal lobe

8.3 Vascular Response in Moyamoya Disease

8.3.1 Autoregulation in Moyamoya Disease

8.3.1.1 Changes in Cerebral Circulation Due to Hyperventilation

Using the ^{133}Xe intracarotid injection method, Uemura et al. [334] found that autoregulation following a rise in blood pressure is well preserved in patients showing no infarctic foci in CT scans. Using our method for continuous measurement of CBF, we have also found that there is almost no increase in rCBF in either the internal carotid arterial system or the vertebrobasilar arterial system

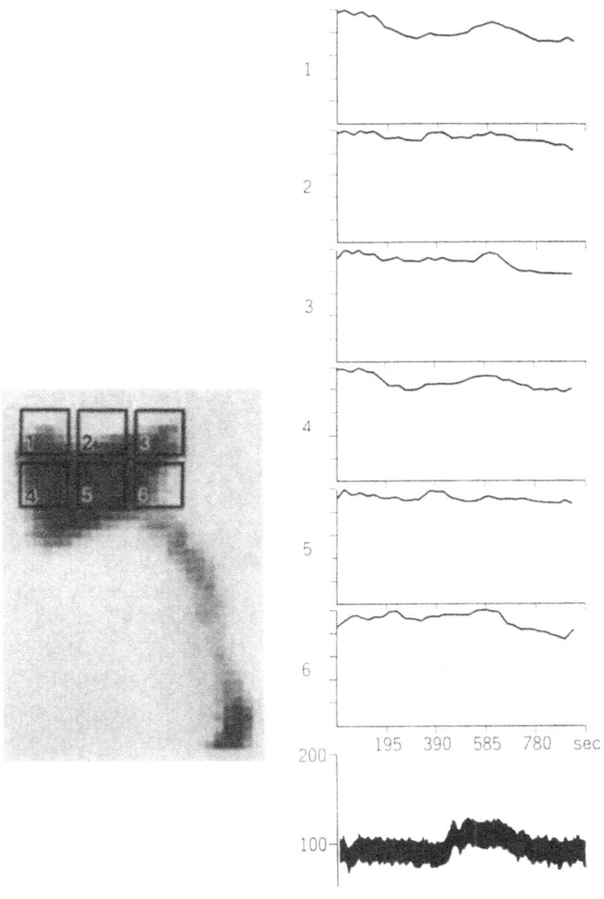

Fig. 85. A 35-year-old male case. Changes in cerebral circulation via the internal carotid arterial system due to hypertension. There is almost no increase in rCBF in any region of interest from 1 to 6 during a rise in blood pressure of 25 mmHg induced by intravenous drip administration of angiotensin II. It is apparent that autoregulation in response to rise in blood pressure is preserved. Change in blood pressure is shown *at the bottom*

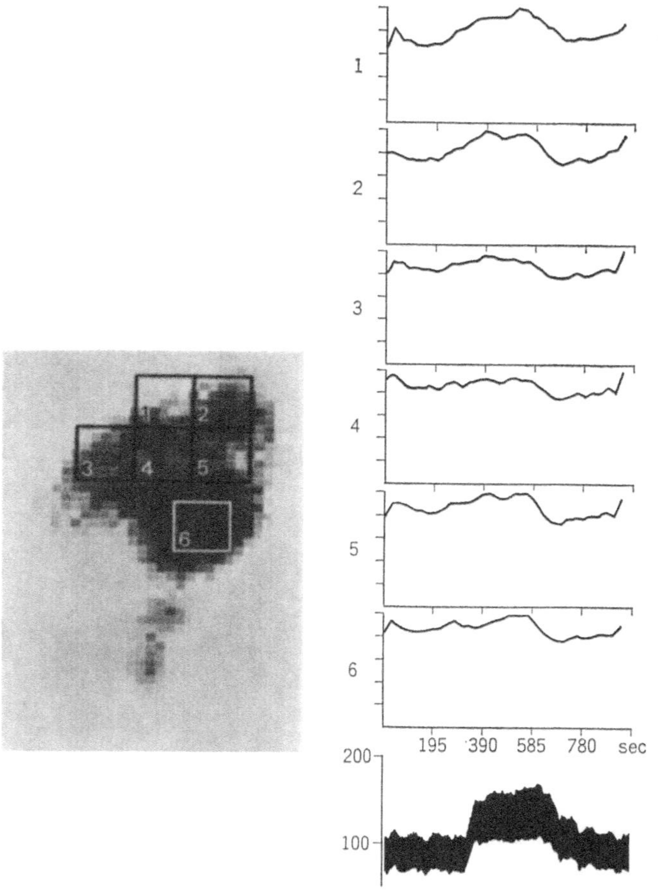

Fig. 86. Changes in cerebral circulation via the vertebrobasilar arterial system due to hypertension in the same case as in Fig. 85. There are only slight increases in rCBF in each region of interest (1–5, posterior half of the cerebrum; 6, cerebellum) during a rise in blood pressure of 50 mmHg induced by intravenous administration of angiotensin II. It is apparent that autoregulation in response to rise in blood pressure is almost preserved. Change in blood pressure is shown *at the bottom*

during a rise in blood pressue of 40 mmHg induced by intravenous administration of angiotensin II (Figs. 85,86). In other words, it is apparent that in moyamoya diseases in which there is no organic damage to the brain autoregulation in response to rises in blood pressure is well preserved.

8.3.1.2 Changes in Cerebral Circulation Due to Hypotension

There have been several studies [215, 328] reporting that there is a tendency for rCBF values to decrease due to the decrease in blood pressure when the head is tilted up. We have induced hypotension by means of intravenous drip of trimetaphan and have found that, in comparison with the change in rCBF induced

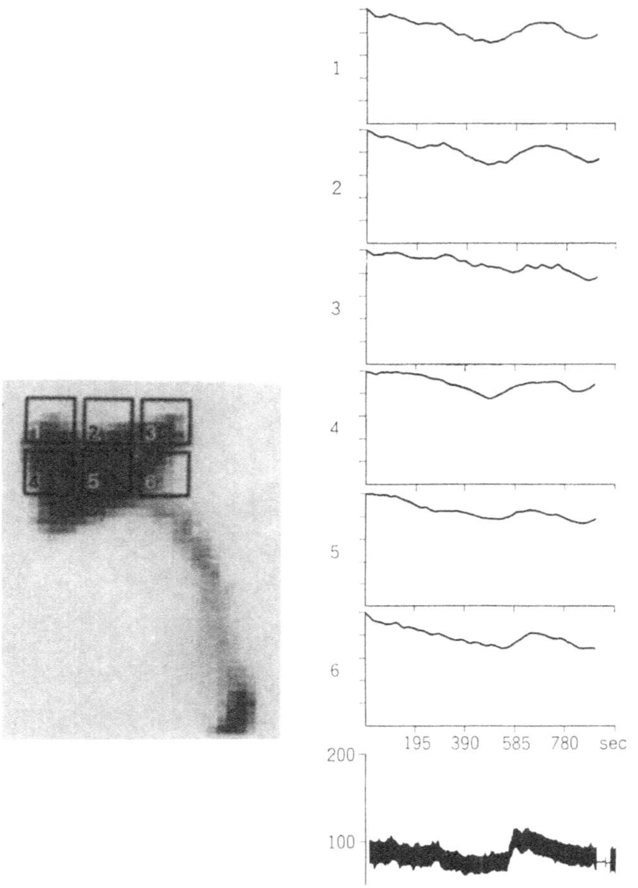

Fig. 87. Changes in cerebral circulation via the internal carotid arterial system due to hypertension in the same case as in Fig. 85. There is a tendency for rCBF values in the regions of interest from 1 to 6 to decrease even during a slight hypotension of 20 mmHg induced by intravenous drip administration of trimetaphane. It is apparent that there is a certain degree of dysautoregulation in response to decrease in blood pressure. Change in blood pressure is shown *at the bottom*

by hypertension, the decreases in both the internal carotid artery and vertebrobasilar artery perfused regions were moderate. However, it should be noted that almost no local differences in the response were found (Figs. 87,88). That is, we believe that even in patients without neurological symptoms there is a certain degree of »dysautoregulation« in response to decreases in blood pressure.

8.3.2 Carbon Dioxide Reactivity

8.3.2.1 Response to CO_2 Inhalation

Using either the nitrous oxide method for measuring the average CBF [303, 328] or the ^{133}Xe intracarotid injection method for measuring rCBF [195, 335], nearly

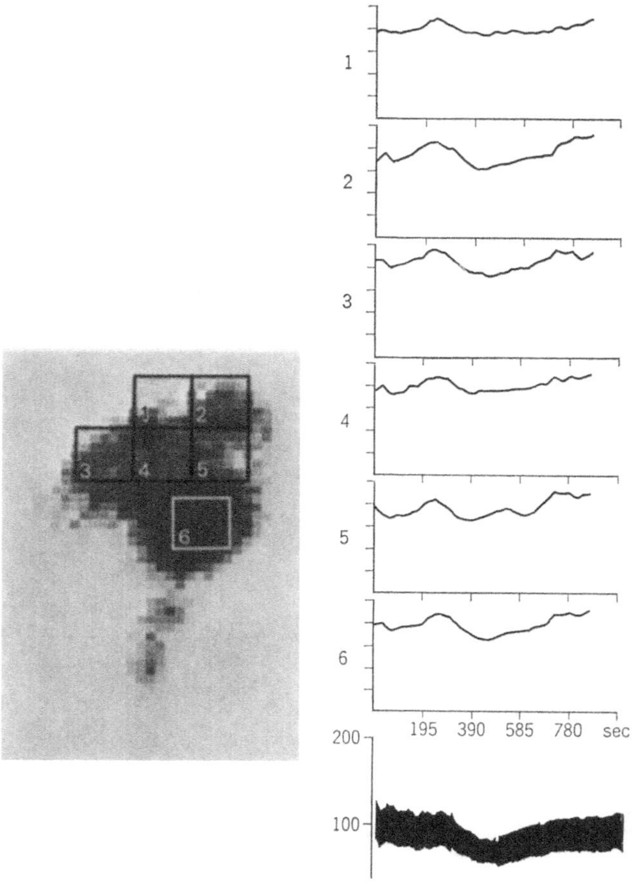

Fig. 88. Changes in cerebral circulation via the vertebrobasilar arterial system due to hypotension in the same case as in Fig. 85. There are changes in rCBF in accordance with the changes in blood pressure (*bottom*) in each region of interest (1–5, posterior half of the cerebrum; 6, cerebellum) during a decrease in blood pressure of 30 mmHg induced by intravenous drip administration of trimetaphane. Autoregulation in response to decrease in blood pressure is disturbed

all cases have shown disturbed CO_2 reactivity. Such disturbances have been severer in juvenile than in adult cases, and there have also been reports that the degree of disturbances varies with location within one and the same patient [180, 215].

We have made an investigation of rCBF changes in internal carotid artery and vertebrobasilar artery perfused areas before and after inhalation of 5% CO_2 using the continuous measurement technique. It was found that, regardless of whether or not there were neurological deficits, only a very small increase in CO_2 reactivity was seen in both areas, as compared with the response seen in normal subjects. These findings suggest that the disturbance of CO_2 reactivity extends to the entire brain, including the cerebellum (Figs. 89, 90).

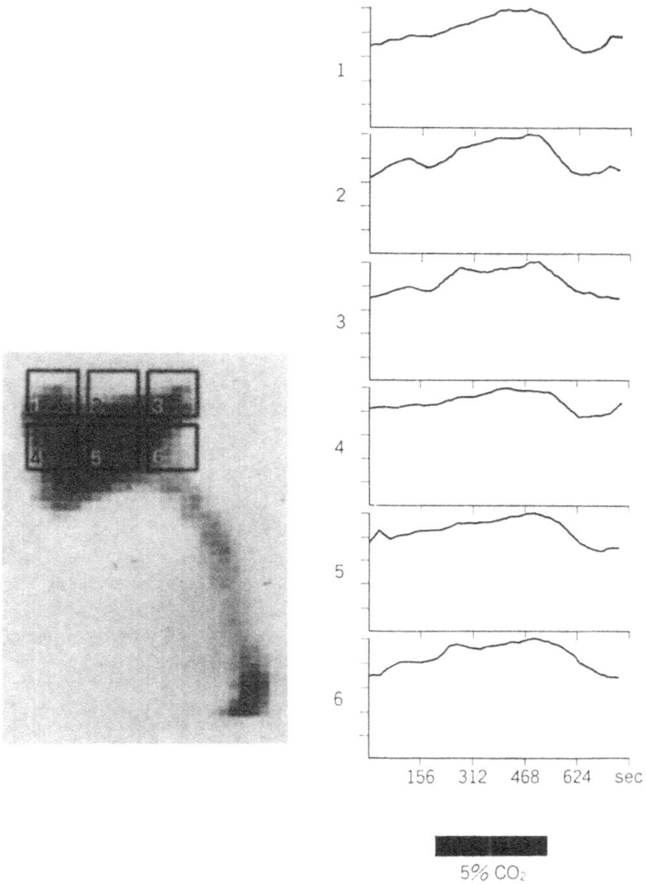

Fig. 89. Carbon dioxide reactivity in the internal carotid artery perfused area in the same case as in Fig. 85. There is a slight increase in rCBF in the regions of interest from 1 to 6 during the inhalation of 5% CO_2; however, the CO_2 reactivity seems weak as compared with the response in normal subjects

8.3.2.2 Response to Hyperventilation

There have been many reports concerned with the changes in cerebral circulation due to hyperventilation in moyamoya disease [217, 328]. All have found that in both adult and children there are decreases in CBF and that such decreases are particularly notable in children. Using the ^{133}Xe intravenous infusion method, we studied the response to hyperventilation in four juvenile and three adult moyamoya cases. In all seven cases there was a decrease in hemispherical blood flow (Fig. 91).

However, Endoh et al. [36] reported a decrease in CBF at sites which are distant from the location of the basal moyamoya vessels themselves. Such results are of particular interest in light of the fact that there appears to be disturbance of the response to hyperventilation at the area of the basal moyamoya vessels.

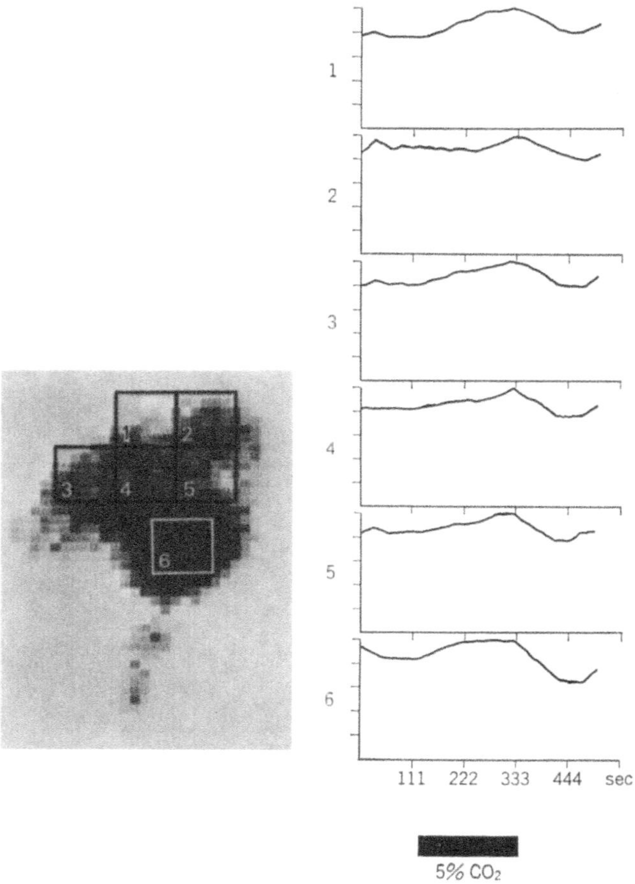

Fig. 90. Carbon dioxide reactivity in the vertebrobasilar artery perfused area in the same case as in Fig. 85. There is a slight increase in rCBF in the regions of interest (1–5, posterior half of the cerebrum; 6, cerebellum) during the inhalation of 5% CO_2; however, the CO_2 reactivity seems weak as compared with the response in normal subjects

Using either the clearance method or the nitrous oxide method, approximately 10 min are required for a single measurement. However, during hyperventilation there are changes with time in the CO_2 and O_2 content of the blood, which means that there may be significant problems in using such measurement techniques. Using a technique for the continuous measurement of CBF in four patients (Table 13), we have found that there is a gradual decrease in blood flow at the area perfused by the vertebrobasilar artery from the start of hyperventilation and that, together with cessation of the hyperventilation, the blood flow increases and returns to the normal preinhalation level within 3–6 min (Fig. 92). In contrast, in the area perfused by the internal carotid artery, there was an increase in rCBF due to hyperventilation and a peak value was recorded at the site of the basal

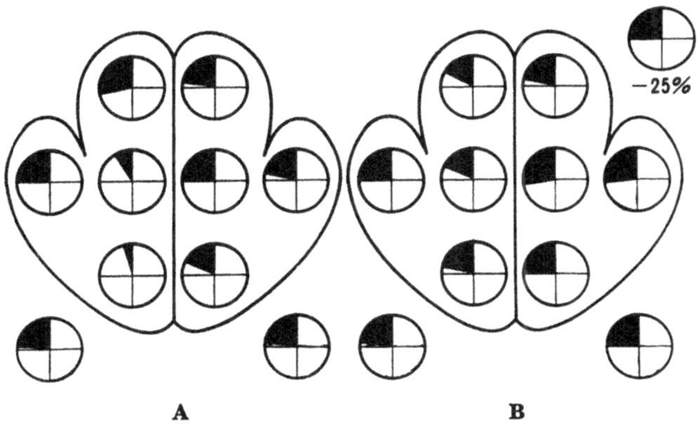

Fig. 91 A, B. Changes in cerebral blood flow due to hyperventilation (^{133}Xe intravenous injection method). There are decreases in rCBF in response to hyperventilation in both adult and juvenile cases. **A** Juvenile cases; **B** adult cases

moyamoya vessels after approximately 4 min of hyperventilation in the juvenile case. In the adult cases, various patterns of changes were found, depending upon the site of measurement (Fig. 93). At some regions, there was a decrease in CBF due to hyperventilation, followed by recovery once hyperventilation had ceased. At other regions, there were no changes due to hyperventilation, but increases in blood flow after hyperventilation. At still other sites, there were virtually no changes during or after hyperventilation.

The fact that, due to hyperventilation, there are regions of the brain at which increases, decreases, or no changes in rCBF are found suggests that the CO_2 reactivity of the vault moyamoya vessels perfused by the external carotid artery may be different from the reactivity of the intracerebral vessels. Differences in reactivity between different parts of the cerebral vascular system could then explain such diverse patterns of blood flow. Definitive answers to such questions are not yet available.

8.4 Conclusion

Summarizing the results obtained by us and others, it can be said that, in adult cases of moyamoya disease which do not show neurological symptoms, the average CBF of the whole brain and hemispheric blood flow is nearly normal. In juvenile cases, it is thought that there are decreases in the whole brain or hemispheric blood flow in comparison with that found in children of comparable ages.

As expected, decreases in rCBF values were observed at the site of organic damage to the brain in both juvenile and adult cases. In cases which did not show neurological symptoms, however, there were increases in blood flow predominantly in the parietal and occipital regions. These findings are thought to

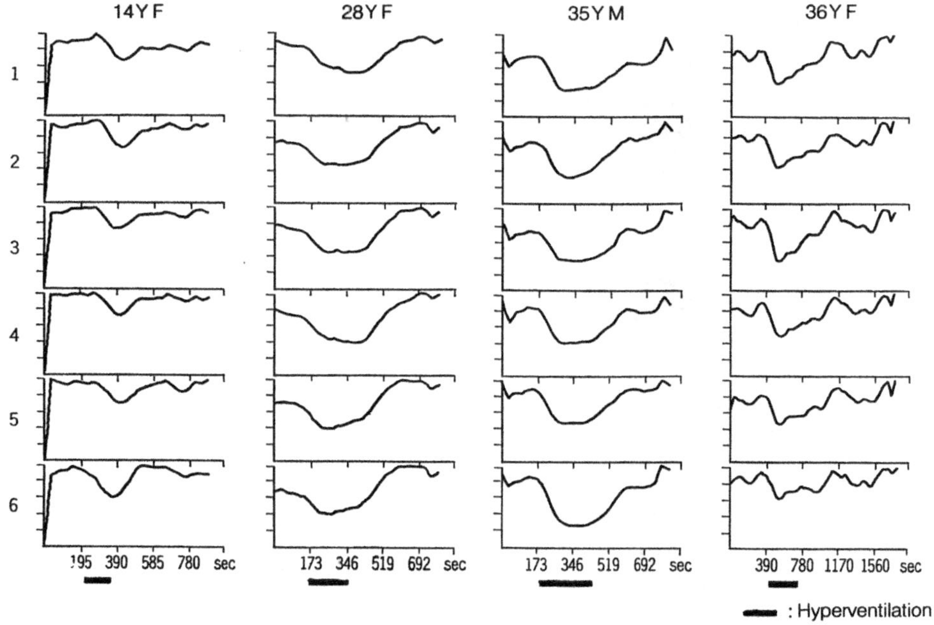

Fig. 92. Changes in cerebral blood flow via the vertebrobasilar arterial system due to hyperventilation. In all cases, there are decreases in rCBF from the start of hyperventilation, and rCBF return to the normal following the cessation of hyperventilation in each region of interest (1–5, posterior half of the cerebrum; 6, cerebellum). The differences in reactivity among the regions were not seen

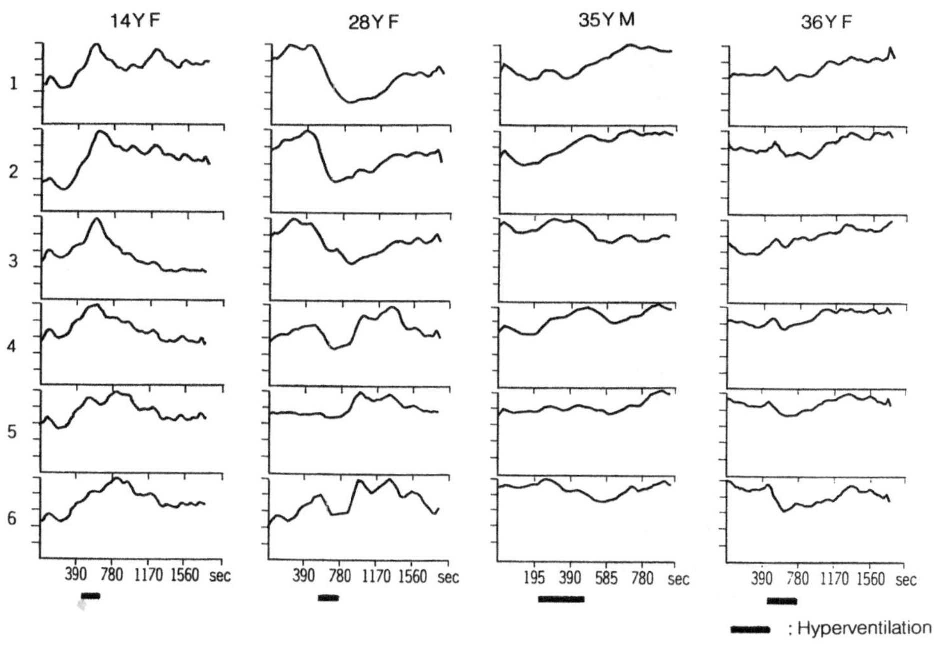

indicate the importance of the collateral pathways via the vertebrobasilar arterial system in moyamoya cases. The blood flow at the site of basal moyamoya was relatively well preserved in all cases, but it was not abnormally high.

With regard to the responsivity of cerebral vessels, autoregulation was preserved in response to rises in blood pressure in most cases, but there were abnormalities of autoregulation in responses to decreases in blood pressure. Although CO_2 reactivity to hyperventilation was generally normal, CO_2 inhalation was disturbed. In other words, in response to loading due to which cerebral vessels normally dilatate, such as CO_2 inhalation or a fall in blood pressure, there are disturbances of the vascular autoregulation in this disease.

Moreover, the differences in vascular responses are thought to be due to slight differences in the nature of the internal carotid arterial and vertebrobasilar arterial systems. The blood supply to the brain in moyamoya disease shows a variety of patterns, including supply via moyamoya vessels from the internal carotid arterial system, supply via ethmoidal moyamoya or vault moyamoya through the external carotid arterial system, or supply through the vertebrobasilar arterial system, and these differences are thought to produce the variety of patterns of vascular responsivity which have been reported in cases of moyamoya disease.

Particularly in juvenile cases of moyamoya disease, this lesion is known to progress and to result in gradual changes in the distribution of cerebral blood flow and vascular responsitivity, together with progression of the disease. We believe that the most enlightening results in future studies will come from detailed follow-up studies of individual cases in which these sequential changes can be studied in detail.

Fig. 93. Changes in cerebral blood flow via the internal carotid arterial system due to hyperventilation. There are some regions where rCBF decreases due to hyperventilation; on the other hand, there are regions where rCBFincreases after the hyperventilation (*1–3*, upper part of the frontal lobe; *4–6*, lower part of the frontal lobe)

9 Treatment

9.1 Introduction

Due to the fact that there are still many uncertainties concerning the pathogenesis of moyamoya disease, thus far no effective and reliable methods for prevention and treatment of this disease have become firmly established. As discussed in the chapter on symptomatology (Chap. 4), in juvenile cases the onset usually presents as symptoms of cerebral ischemia due to repeated transient ischemic attacks (TIAs). The disease gradually progresses and at a certain stage the symptoms of brain ischemia disappear. At the next stage, there are many adult cases which manifest symptoms of intracranial hemorrhage, particularly intraventricular hemorrhage [133, 284]. For treatment of such pathology, various methods for increasing blood flow to the brain via collateral pathways have been attempted and, to reduce the effects of the hemorrhage itself, various techniques for hematoma removal have been attempted.

On the basis of various research findings, we have suspected that the cervical sympathetic nerves are critically involved in the development of moyamoya disease. We have consequently performed superior cervical ganglionectomy (SCGectomy) and perivascular sympathectomy (PVSectomy) at the cervical portion of the internal carotid artery (ICA) and have thereby obtained relatively favorable therapeutic results. In this chapter, this and other therapeutic steps currently in use for therapy in cases of moyamoya disease are discussed, including STA-MCA anastomosis, which has been a principal therapeutic method.

9.2 Therapy of Infarction Attacks

9.2.1 Drug Treatment

Steroid hormones and antibiotics have been administered in some cases, but suppression of the progress of the disease has not been achieved. Although administration of vasodilators or drugs with facilitatory effects on cerebral blood flow has been attempted and, although, immediately following onset of symptoms due to brain ischemia, various conservative treatments have been pursued (such as administration of mannitol, low molecular weight dextran, anesthetic blockers to the cervical sympathetics, or cerebral metabolic activators), improvements in symptoms have not been obtained.

At the time of TIA-like symptoms, however, it is known that a rise in $PaCO_2$ brought about simply by placing a plastic bag over the patient's head will allow the attack to pass mildly [356]. This method can produce good effects for temporary alleviation of symptoms, but the patient's respiratory condition should be observed closely when using this technique.

9.2.2 Surgical Treatment

9.2.2.1 Durapexia

In 1964, Tsubokawa and colleagues [331] reported on the treatment of the case of 6-year-old child thought probably to be moyamoya disease. Their surgical technique included placing a portion of the dura mater, including the middle meningeal artery (MMA), on the surface of the brain. They reported that angiograms taken 2 months postoperatively showed formation of collateral pathways to the arteries of the surface of the brain via the middle meningeal artery and that symptoms had improved. Unfortunately, no further reports concerning this therapeutic technique have appeared since then.

9.2.2.2 Cervical Perivascular Sympathectomy (PVSectomy) and Superior Cervical Ganglionectomy (SCGectomy)

In previous studies, we have demonstrated that there are sympathetic nerve fibers reaching the walls of the arteries of the human brain down to the size of arterioles, and that they are particularly abundant in the arteries around the circle of Willis [260]. Moreover, in animal experiments, we have shown that the sympathetic nerve endings within the arterioles of the intracranial internal carotid arterial system originate in the superior cervical ganglion [299]. Since these sympathetic fibers which are distributed to such vascular walls have vasoconstrictive effects, we surmised that cervical PVSectomy [271] and SCGectomy [294] would result in the dilatation of the vessels of the internal and external carotid arterial systems, increase blood flow along collateral pathways, and therefore constitute a therapeutic technique for cerebral circulatory insufficiency.

We have reported elsewhere [238, 295] that this method can be used with good results for alleviation of symptoms of cerebral infarction due to vasospasm following aneurysm rupture. Furthermore, complications are extremely rare using this technique.

Among our 100 cases of moyamoya disease, this therapeutic technique has been used in 31 juvenile cases (less than 15 years of age) and 17 adult cases, all with symptoms of cerebral ischemia. However, these 48 cases include cases which were operated on unilaterally or upon whom SCGectomy alone was performed. Thus far, a total of 21 juvenile cases and 10 adult cases have had both PVSectomy and SCGectomy performed bilaterally, and in recent cases this bilateral complete operation has been performed in all cases regardless of the stage of the moyamoya disease. The results produced using this technique are noteworthy and will be discussed in detail below. Moreover, we have performed follow-up studies (ranging from 6 months to 14 years postoperatively) and investigated the changes in symptoms and intelligence between the preoperative and postoperative periods. Among those, angiographical follow-up has been possible in nine juvenile cases for postoperative periods ranging from 1 to 14 years.

Surgical Method (Fig. 94). With the patient's head titled slightly contralaterally, the cervical region is somewhat extended and a descending 60-mm skin incision is made from slightly above the height of the mandibular angle after tracing the anteromedial edge of the sternocleidomastoid muscle. That muscle is then pushed externally.

The common carotid artery and the bifurcation of the internal carotid artery and external carotid artery are then exposed. Perivascular denervation is easily accomplished, provided that a wheal is made between the adventitia and media by saline injection. The PVSectomy is performed in the entire region, approximately 10 mm below the carotid bifurcation and over a length of approximately 10 mm along the internal carotid artery. It is known that the superior cervical ganglion is present at a site somewhat rostromedioposterior from the bifurcation of the internal and external carotid arteries and on the longus capitus muscle, but it can sometimes be difficult to find. However, provided that one has a good conception of the local topography in mind, the sympathetic trunk nerves can always be discovered by searching in this vicinity. By following the trunk nerves rostrally, the superior cervical ganglion will be discovered.

The communicating branches of this ganglion are severed as far as possible and the entire ganglion is removed. During this procedure, it is inevitable that some pressure is put on the internal carotid artery in the medial direction, but pressure

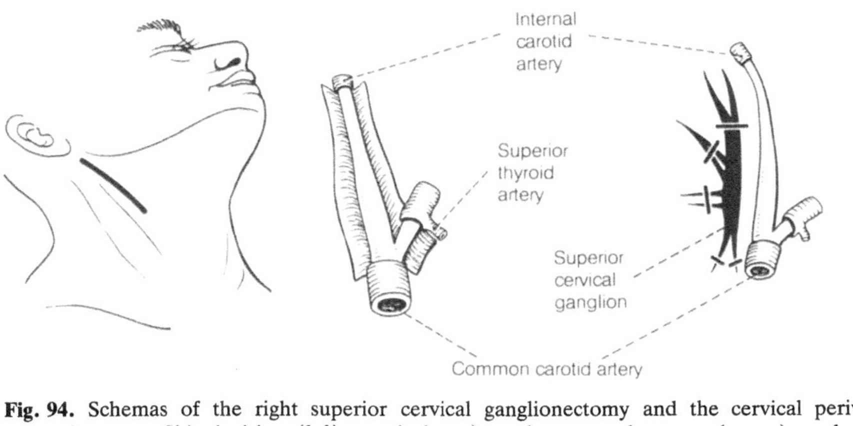

Fig. 94. Schemas of the right superior cervical ganglionectomy and the cervical perivascular sympathectomy. Skin incision (*left*), cervical perivascular sympathectomy (*center*), and superior cervical ganglionectomy (*right*)

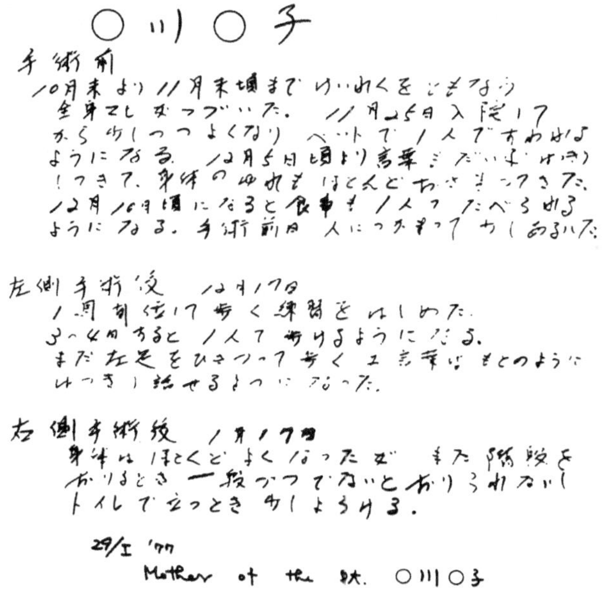
○川○子
手術前
10月末より11月末頃までけいれんをともなう
全身マヒがつづいた。11月25日入院して
から少しづつよくなりベットで1人ですわれる
ようになる。12月5日頃より言葉がだいぶはっきり
してきて、身体のゆれもほとんどなくなってきた。
12月16日頃になると食事も1人でたべられる
ようになる。手術前日人につかまって少し歩いた

左側手術後 12月17日
1週間位して歩く練習をはじめた。
3～4日すると1人で歩けるようになる。
まだ左足をひきずって歩く。言葉はもとのように
はっきり話せるようになった。

右側手術後 1月17日
身体はほとんどよくなったが、また階段を
おりるとき一段づつでないとおりられない
トイレで立つとき少しよろける。

29/I '77
Mother of the pt. ○川○子

Before the operation:
General motor weakness, sometimes combined with convulsions, had persisted from October to November. After she was admitted to hospital on November 25th, her condition improved and she was able to sit on the bed without support. Around December 5th, her speech become clearer and the instability of her body improved.
On December 10th, she could take a meal without help and walked a little with assistance.

After the operation on the left side (December 17th):
About a week later she started practicing walking and she could walk by herself 3 to 4 days after. She dragged her left leg, but her speech became as clear as before.

After the operation on the right side (January 17th):
She looked almost normal: however, she could only go down the stairs one step at a time and was still unsteady when standing up in the bathroom.

Fig. 95. The records of pre- and postoperative symptoms of a patient written by the patient's family

such that this vessel becomes occluded should be avoided. Moreover, care must be taken not to bring about damage to the vagus or the hypoglossal nerves.

Such perivascular denervation cannot be performed bilaterally in a single operation; at least 2 weeks recovery time should be allowed following unilateral denervation before contralateral operation is attempted.

Follow-up of Clinical Symptoms. Follow-up of clinical symptoms after surgical treatment in our cases was carried out primarily by means of collecting the observations of the parents and immediate family concerning the patient's condition [114] (Fig. 95). Among our 31 cases, 19 (61.3%) showed improvement of clinical symptoms, 9 remained unchanged, and 3 showed deterioration (Table 14).

Table 14. Surgical treatment for juvenile cases. Improvement of clinical symptoms was observed in 19 out of 31 cases (61.3 %)

Operation	Results			Total
	Improved	Unchanged	Aggravated	
Bilateral PVS	1	2	1	4
Unilateral PVS and contralateral PVS + SCG	3	3	0	6
Bilateral PVS + SCG	15	4	2	21
Total	19(61,3 %)	9(29.0 %)	3(9,7 %)	31

PSV, perivascular sympathectomy; SCG, superior cervical ganglionectomy

Table 15. Surgical treatment for adults cases. Improvement of clinical symptoms was observed in 8 out of 17 cases (47.1 %)

Operation	Results			Total
	Improved	Unchanged	Aggravated	
Bilateral PVS	1	0	0	4
Unilateral PVS and contralateral PVS + SCG	1	2	0	3
Bilateral PVS + SCG	3	7	0	10
Total	8(47,1 %)	9(52,9 %)	0(0 %)	17

Among the 21 juvenile cases in which PVSectomy and SCGectomy were performed bilaterally, improvement was seen in 15 (74%), no change in 4, and deterioration in 2. Among the 17 adult cases, 8 (47.1%) showed improvement of clinical symptoms and the remaining 9 showed no change (Table 15).

With regard to the change in the symptoms, the following results were obtained. Among the juvenile cases, 16 of the 26 who had shown TIA-like symptoms had complete disappearance of such attacks. Among the 16 who had bilateral PVSectomy and SCGectomy, such attacks disappeared in 12 and were reduced in frequency in 4. All of the eight cases who had shown involuntary movements showed disappearance of such symptoms. Among the 17 cases who

Table 16. Result of surgical treatment in juvenile cases

Symptom	Presurgery	Follow-up
Episode of TIA	26 cases	→ 16 No episode
		→ 7 Improved
		→ 3 Worsened
Involuntary movement	8	→ 8 Cured
Mental handicap	17	
Educationable (50<IQ<80)	11	→ 1 Normal range
		→ 8 Improved
		→ 2 Stationary
Uneducationable (IQ<50)	6	→ 6 Stationary

Table 17. Result of surgical treatment in adult cases

Symptom	Presurgery	Follow-up
Motor disturbance	8 cases	→ 5 Improved → 4 Stationary
Sensory disturbance	3	→ 3 Stationary
Speech disturbance	4	→ 3 Improved → 1 Stationary
Visual disturbance	4	→ 2 Improved → 2 Stationary
Mental handicap	9	→ 4 Improved → 5 Stationary

had shown deficits of intelligence, 1 of the 11 mild cases showed return of IQ to a normal range and 8 showed some improvement, but among the cases with IQs below 50 there were no improvements (Table 16). Among the adult cases, improvements were seen in five of the nine cases with motor disturbances, in three of the four with speech disturbances, in two of the four with visual acuity abnormalities, and in four of the nine with psychic disturbances. None of these patients showed deterioration (Table 17). In other words, in nearly all of the patients there were some improvements in the symptoms of moyamoya disease. Moreover, such improvements were seen in the early postoperative period and continued thereafter. The majority of the cases showing improvements were those which had had bilateral PVSectomy and SCGectomy performed, and most of those not showing improvements had had incomplete or unilateral surgical treatment. As is apparent from the above, this therapeutic method is effective and the degree of improvement is similar to that seen following STA-MCA anastomosis, to be described below. Since the PVSectomy and SCGectomy techniques are not intracranial operations, complications are few and we consequently consider this method to be the first choice in the surgical treatment of moyamoya disease.

There were, in fact, three cases in which there was postoperative deterioration of symptoms. One showed a marked decrease in blood pressure during the operation, and the other two might have had marked decreases in cerebral blood flow due to compression of the internal carotid artery during the surgical operation. Therefore it is believed that maintenance of normal levels of blood flow to the brain is extremely important when using this technique.

Angiographic Follow-up. Angiographic follow-up was made within 2 months from surgery on 13 sides in 9 subjects. Eight sides showed angiographical improvement – that is, increases in basal moyamoya, the appearance of cerebral main trunk arteries, dilatation of the terminal portion of the internal carotid artery, etc. However, three sides were unchanged and two showed deterioration based upon the six-stage classification of moyamoya disease [287] (see Chap. 3). In contrast, among the ten sides in six cases followed up 6 months after surgery, eight sides showed progression of the moyamoya disease, as determined by the above-mentioned classification, and two were unchanged. In other words, angiographically, such therapy was found to be effective for only a short period of about 2 months [294].

Although the results of the continued improvements in clinical symptoms and the progression of the disease, as seen angiographically, appear at first glance to be contradictory, it is thought that PVSectomy and SCGectomy therapy results in increases in collateral blood flow to the brain via routes other than the basal moyamoya, i.e., via the external carotid arterial system and the vertebrobasilar arterial system.

9.3 Superficial Temporal Artery-Cortical Branch of the Middle Cerebral Artery Anastomosis (STA-MCA Anastomosis) and Encephalomyosynangiosis

The STA-MCA anastomosis technique, which was developed in 1967 by Yasargil et al. for treatment of ischemic cerebrovascular disorders, was first used for treatment of moyamoya disease in 1974 by Krayenbühl [140], Karasawa [108] and Kikuchi [108, 121]. Unlike most other ischemic cerebrovascular disorders, however, in moyamoya disease the recipient arteries at the surface of the brain are small and narrow.

Consequently, for those cases which do not have an appropriate recipient artery, Kikuchi et al. introduced an operative technique called encephalomyosynangiosis (EMS) [70], in which a portion of temporal muscle is attached to the surface of the brain [106]. They have since used one or both of these surgical techniques in the treatment of 37 cases (through 1979) [4, 12, 18, 19, 107, 112, 117, 138, 197, 274]. They have reported that in postoperative selective external carotid angiograms, in addition to visualization of the middle cerebral artery due to anastomosis, they also find spontaneous anastomosis of the dural arteries and, moreover, in many cases there has been visualization of cortical branches of the middle cerebral artery through newly developed moyamoya vessels at the surface of the brain. In contrast, carotid angiograms revealed that there were fewer moyamoya vessels and that the middle cerebral arteries were poorly visualized as compared with the preoperative state, or that in some cases there was even a complete failure to visualize the middle cerebral artery. As for clinical symptoms, there were cases of disappearance or improvement of ischemic symptoms of the middle cerebral artery and disappearance or reduction of transient ischemic attacks in 35 cases, and no changes in only 2 cases.

In addition, follow-up of 29 cases more than 3½ years after surgery showed marked therapeutic effectiveness for ischemic symptoms of the MCA, although no effectiveness was found for visual acuity disturbances, homonymous hemianopsia or swallowing disturbances.

The effectiveness of such therapy has since been reported by others as well [128, 197, 199, 352] and it is now thought that these are the most common surgical techniques used in Japan for moyamoya disease. There are, however, some reports of aggravation of neurological symptoms and of other complications [199, 274, 318] and we have experienced the cases of postoperative bilateral paralysis, speech disturbances, and mental deterioration in which this surgical therapy has been performed at other clinics. These results lead us to believe that further study of these surgical techniques is required.

9.4 Transplantation of the Omentum

Transplantation of the omentum involves resection of the omentum, including the gastroepiploic artery and vein and anastomosis of these vessels to the superficial temporal artery and vein, leaving the omentum on the surface of the brain [349, 351]. This technique has been applied by Karasawa et al. [109] and Yonekawa and Handa [352] in cases of moyamoya disease. The omentum covers a larger portion of the surface of the brain than the temporal muscle piece (and should therefore allow for the development of relatively more collateral pathways to the brain), but meaningful evaluation of this method is still not possible due to the extremely small number of clinical cases treated thus far.

9.5 Encephaloduroarteriosynangiosis

In 1980, Matsushima et al. [173] introduced a method in which the dura mater was cut linearly and the arteries of the scalp (the superficial temporal artery or the occipital artery) were exposed with subjacent fascia. Without cutting the peripheral end of these vessels, suturing of the dura mater with fascia including artery through a long and narrow bone window was attempted in a 9-year-old moyamoya case. Six months later, angiographically, fine collateral vessels to the brain surface were seen. Neurological symptoms improved and Matsushima et al. have argued that this technique is either superior to or as good as EMS or STA-MCA anastomosis. Among the advantages of this technique is the fact that the surgical technique itself is not difficult, there is no need to sacrifice the EC-IC anastomosis which is present prior to surgery (transdural anastomosis — vault moyamoya) [135], and no invasion of the brain tissue is required. That is, compression of the brain, temporary vascular occlusion, and/or relative increases in the weight of the brain due to aspiration of cerebrospinal fluid are not brought about. Consequently, there are few deleterious effects on cerebral blood flow during the operation. It is believed therefore, that the complications sometimes seen with STA-MCA anastomosis, etc. will be infrequent. Moreover, there is the advantage that the anterior and posterior branches of the STA, the occipital artery, and other arteries over the brain surface can be used as the donor arteries. Since 1980, Matsushima et al. have used this technique in nine cases of childhood moyamoya disease (13 sides) [174]. Angiographically, revascularization of the vessels of the brain surface from the donor artery was seen, together with gradual disappearance of the moyamoya vessels at the base of the brain.

In addition to the above methods, ligation of the peripheral end of the transected STA, which is then left of the surface of the brain (encephaloarteriosynangiosis) [197], has been reported. The development of collateral pathways to the brain surface have then been found to arise. Since the brain in moyamoya disease is in a state of chronic ischemia and there is therefore thought to be a demand for blood from whatever source [15, 197, 275], these surgical techniques are thought to be responsible for the acceleration of revascularization. However, considerable time is required for the development of such revascularization and there is inevitably adhesion with the brain surface. Due to even extremely mild trauma, it is possible that hemorrhage could occur at that site and an epileptic focus could develop.

We currently believe that the best therapeutic technique is a combination of PVSectomy and SCGectomy, with their immediate effects, and Matsushima's encephaloduroarteriosynangiosis with its delayed effects.

9.6 Therapy for and Prevention of Intracranial Hemorrhage

The intracranial hemorrhage which is seen in some 4% of juvenile cases and some 50%–80% of adult cases [310] is generally understood to be subarachnoid hemorrhage from the nature of the manifesting symptoms. Nonetheless, since before the widespread usage of CT scanning, we have emphasized the fact that a large majority of the intracranial bleedings have their source in the vicinity of the superior lateral wall of the lateral ventricle – most of which penetrate into the lateral ventricles, causing intraventricular hemorrhage. Recently, the truth of this assertion has been demonstrated in both CT and autopsy studies. Moreover, as mentioned earlier, saccular aneurysm of the basilar artery easily develops in moyamoya disease, but it is known that genuine subarachnoid hemorrhage due to its rupture is in fact rare. Consequently, in the therapy of intracranial hemorrhage, appropriate therapy is undertaken in accordance with the current therapy for the intracranial hematoma, the intraventricular hematoma, and/or the aneurysm [12, 71, 80, 266].

Next a few cases of our own are presented.

Case 1: 51-year-old Female

Anamnesis: In 1972, this patient experienced ten continuous days of unconsciousness, during which lumber puncture showed bloody cerebrospinal fluid. Angiography led to a diagnosis of moyamoya disease.

Present illness: On 28 February 1982, she experienced headache, vomiting, and left hemiparesis and was immediately hospitalized. CTscans showed intracerebral hematoma in the right frontal lobe and ventricular penetration (Fig. 74). Carotid angiograms revealed the moyamoya disease. An emergency operation was performed on that day. The intracerebral hematoma was removed, the intraventricular hematoma was removed from the anterior horn of both lateral ventricles, and continuous ventricular drainage was instituted. About 60 g hematoma was aspirated. The postoperative course has been favorable and she is now undergoing rehabilitation for the left paresis. Nearly all of the hemorrhage in this case was intracerebral, with penetration into the ventricle being slight.

Case 2: A 49-year-old Male

Anamnesis: In 1977, this patient presented symptoms of cerebral ischemia and was diagnosed as having moyamoya disease.

Present illness: On 27 November 1979, he experienced sudden severe headache and loss of consciousness and was hospitalized at our clinic. He was comatose on

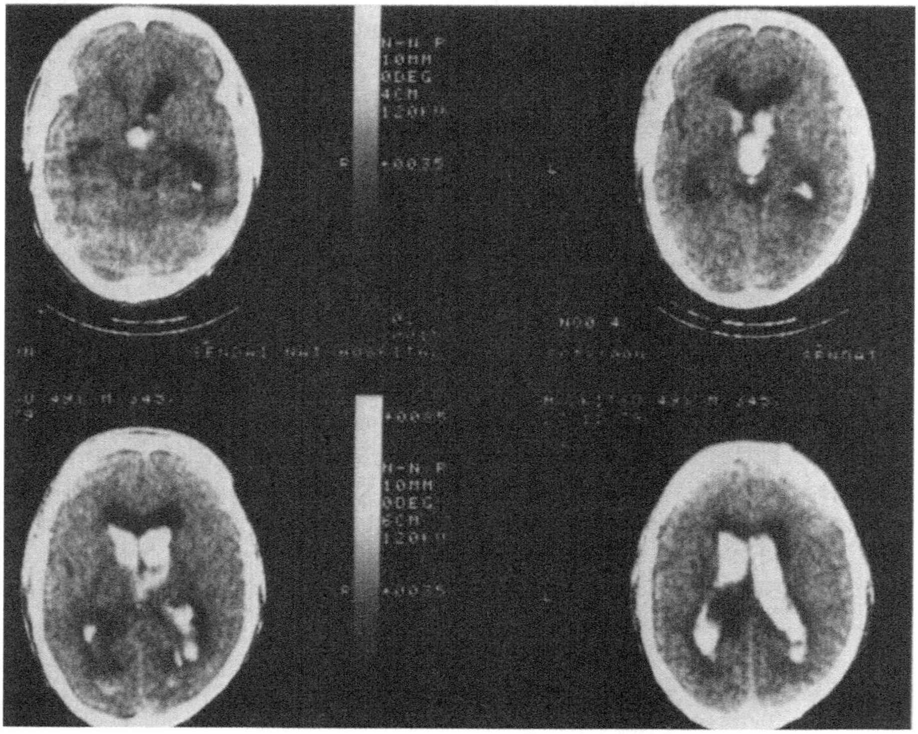

Fig. 96. A 49-year-old male case. CT scan taken on emergent admission showed intraventricular hematoma filling bilateral lateral ventricles

admission, but there was no paresis of the limbs and subarachnoid hemorrhage was suspected. CT scans (Fig. 96), however, showed the lateral ventricles to be filled with a hematoma. Extirpation of the ventricular hematoma from the anterior horn to the posterior horn was performed bilaterally, followed by institution of continuous ventricular drainage. Postoperatively, consciousness gradually returned to normal and after 65 days in hospital he was discharged capable of normal daily activities.

In the extirpation of such hematomas which fill the ventricles like a mold in a cast, it is necessary to make burr holes bilaterally at the top of the forehead and, furthermore, to consider that the direction of the ventricular puncture is parallel to the trunk of the lateral ventricle. By going in this direction, it is possible to excise the entire hematoma from the anterior to the posterior horn [202] (Fig. 97). After hematoma removal, a large ventricular drainage tube is inserted bilaterally and the tip of the tube is placed not in the posterior horn or body of the ventricle, but in the anterior horn. In this way, the obstruction of the drainage tube by blood clots can be reduced and a few days later the drainage tube can be removed. If high intracranial pressure prevents this, however, a shunt operation should be undertaken. As in the present case, where there was almost no intracerebral hematoma, but rather an entirely intraventricular hematoma, if competent surgical treatment is done within an appropriate period, the prognosis will be good.

Since the intracranial and intraventricular hemorrhage seen in this patient was brought about by the above-mentioned mechanism, it requires lifelong control of blood pressure, as is the case in hypertensive intracerebral hemorrhage. Moyamoya disease is, however, fundamentally a disease of cerebral ischemia, so that excessive hypotension would again bring about symptoms due to brain ischemia. The control of the hypertension must be well understood and carefully undertaken, and we believe that capillary stabilizers should also be used.

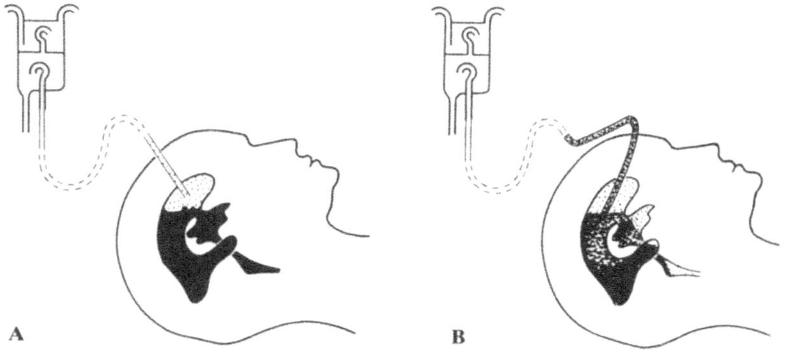

Fig. 97 A, B. Comparison between the current method of ventricular drainage (**A**) and the method of removal of intraventricular hematoma by our continuous ventricular drainage (**B**). It is possible to remove more intraventricular hematoma with the latter method

9.7 Anesthesia During Surgery for Moyamoya Disease

It is known that cerebral ischemia can be produced in moyamoya disease due to hyperventilation. Moreover, the brain in moyamoya disease is in a state of chronic ischemia, so that a fall in cerebral perfusion which is produced by a fall in systemic blood pressure due to anesthetic can cause aggravation of symptoms postoperatively. Consequently, hyperventilation and a fall in systemic blood pressure during anesthesia must be avoided.

Kuro et al. [152] selected the $PaCO_2$ of blood from the jugular bulbus as an index of cerebral blood flow and investigated the relationship between $PaCO_2$, systemic blood pressure, and cerebral blood flow. They found that $PaCO_2$ was closely related to changes in cerebral blood flow. During mNLA (modified neuroleptoanalgesia) anesthesia, $PaCO_2$ was 30 mmHg, while during GOF (nitrogen dioxide, oxygen, halothane) anesthesia it was below 25 mmHg, leading to cerebral ischemia. They pointed out that in using either anesthetic, $PaCO_2$ should be maintained at about 45 mmHg. Moreover, the effects of GOF anesthesia on cerebral autoregulation were strong, indicating the necessity of avoiding hypotension. Consequently, when undertaking surgical treatment in cases of moyamoya disease, it is essential that sufficient systemic blood pressure be maintained and, by means of frequent checks of blood gases, the decrease in $PaCO_2$ be closely monitored.

9.8 Conclusion

The natural course of moyamoya disease results in recurring mild deficits in most cases. Particularly in juvenile cases, progressive aggravation occurs in some 30% and mild deficits in 30%, so that more than one-half of juvenile cases of moyamoya disease have lasting neurological deficits. A relatively small number of children are capable of returning to fully normal social lives. We believe that in the evaluation of the therapeutic effects in moyamoya disease, comparison with the results when the disease is allowed to follow its natural course is important.

In the 48 cases showing symptoms of cerebral ischemia, for which PVSectomy and SCGectomy have been performed since 1963, long-term follow-up has not revealed any notable undesirable side effects. Nineteen of the 31 juvenile cases (61.3%) and 8 of the 17 adult cases (41.1%) showed improvement of symptoms. Particularly among the 21 juvenile cases in which bilateral operations were performed, 15 (17.4%) showed improvement, suggesting that quite reliable, if less than perfect, therapeutic effects can be obtained using this method. The fact that the rate of effectiveness was favorable among juvenile cases is thought to be due to the fact that the capacity for developing collateral pathways is greater than in adult cases. Since the surgical technique is not difficult and, provided that a fall in cerebral blood flow due to the anesthetic is avoided as mentioned above, this therapeutic technique is thought to be relatively safe, as well.

In recent years, various intracranial techniques, such as STA-MCA anastomosis, EMS, and EDAS (encephaloduroarteriosynangiosis) have been devised, and there are many reports of favorable surgical results using those techniques. It cannot be said, however, that STA-MCA anastomosis is always a safe technique, as discussed above. In addition, although the EMS techniques were developed because of the problems of finding an appropriate recipient artery, it involves adhesion between a portion of temporal muscle, fascia or dura mater, and the surface of the brain to allow for the development of collateral pathways. This region of adhesion is widespread and, consequently, there is remaining concern that this could become an epileptic focus subsequently or that the adhesion could be torn due to slight trauma and that the damage to the brain tissue could be the source of intracranial hemorrhage. Furthermore, in such treatment, in order to perform the required large craniotomy, the superficial temporal artery or middle meningeal artery (which will be the feeding artery of the vault moyamoya seen in the calotte) must be cut, and this could actually lead to a decrease in cerebral blood flow.

We have found that quite effective results are obtained when PVSectomy and SCGectomy were performed on both sides, with each side treated several weeks apart. The advantages of this technique are that the surgical method is relatively simple, no intracranial invasion is required, and side effects are uncommon. Although effectiveness cannot be expected in cases with severe deficits of intelligence, if the above-mentioned precautions are taken, PVSectomy and SCGectomy together are thought to be the first choice for surgical treatment. Moreover, the EDAS method developed by Matsushima et al. allows for the accelerated development of collateral pathways, but does not require invasion of the brain tissue. We believe that, in conjunction with our method, these two techniques constitute a safer and more effective means of treating moyamoya disease.

10 Pathology

10.1 Introduction

Many autopsy studies have been made on stenotic changes at the terminal portion of the internal carotid artery, which are known to be the initial cause of moyamoya disease. Nonetheless, the essential nature of the pathology involved has remained unclear. This unsatisfactory situation with regard to our understanding of the pathology of moyamoya disease has prompted us to make a study of the findings from all of those autopsy studies reported over the past 20 years.

10.2. Autopsy Materials

Materials for the present investigation included 10 autopsy cases studied by us [193, 292] and 61 cases reported in the literature [2, 5, 6, 16, 22, 23, 37, 45, 56, 59, 61, 76, 78, 81–86, 101, 102, 120, 122, 165, 167, 175, 225, 226, 229, 231, 256, 270, 321, 322, 339]. These 71 cases are summarized in Table 18 and Fig. 98.

A total of 10 juvenile cases (3 male, 7 female) have been reported; the remaining 61 cases (24 male, 37 female) were 16 years of age or older. A slight

Table 18. Pathological findings of our ten autopsy cases

	Case No.	Age	Sex	Past history	Pathological findings
Juvenile cases	1	4	F	Measles	Cerebral infarction
	2[a]	7	M	(−)	Cerebral infarction, stenotic change of renal artery
Adult cases	3	31	M	Sinusitis	ICH (putamen), IVH
	4	48	F	Hypertension	ICH (putamen), IVH
	5	36	F	Cerebral palsy	ICH (putamen), IVH
	6	41	F	(−)	ICH (thalamus), IVH, nonruptured basilar aneurysm
	7	33	F	(−)	ICH (thalamus), IVH
	8	19	F	TIA	ICH (claustrum), IVH
	9	34	F	Tonsilitis	Cerebral infarction
	10[a]	37	F	Nephritis, hypertension	Cerebral infarction, stenotic of renal artery, coronary artery and aorta

ICH, intracerebral hemorrhage; IVH, intraventricular hemorrhage; TIA, transient ischemic attack
[a] Whole body autopsy

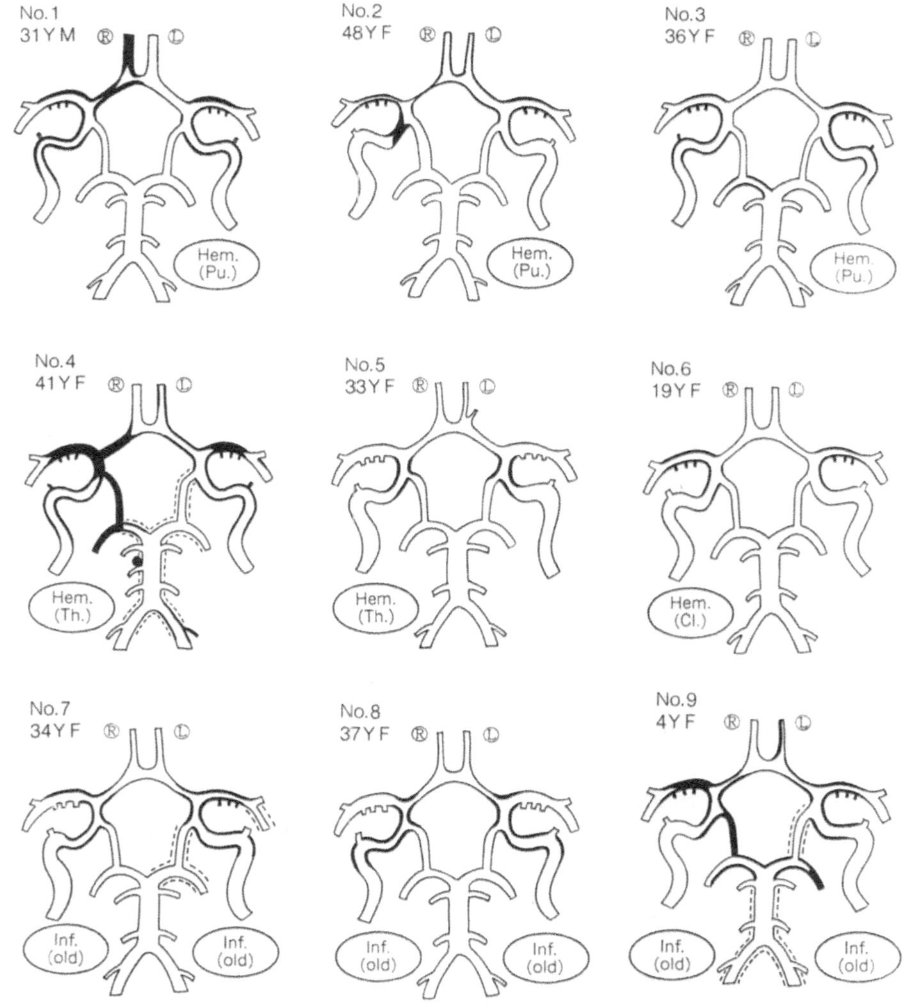

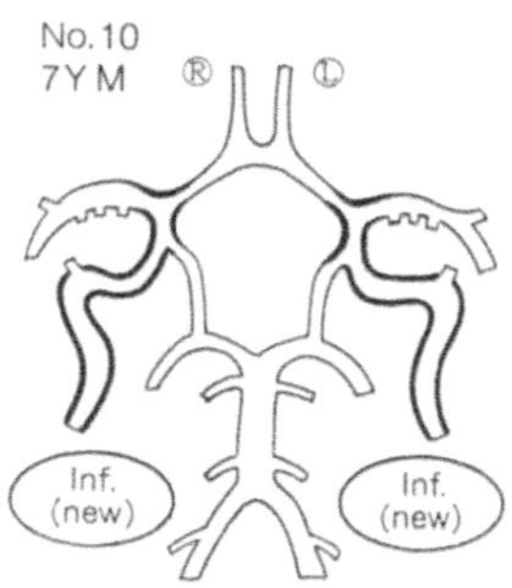

Fig. 98. Schemas of the main cerebral arteries at the base of the brain of our ten autopsied cases, showing stenotic or occluded portions. *Hem. (Pu.)*, putaminal hemorrhage; *Hem. (Th.)*, thalamic hemorrhage; *Hem. (Cl.)*, claustral hemorrhage; *Inf. (old)*, obsolete infarction; *Inf. (new)*, fresh infarction. *Thick lines* show stenotic or occluded portions due to intimal thickening and *dotted lines* show dilated portions due to medial thickening

preponderance of female cases relative to male cases was found (44:27). It has not been possible to determine the cause of death in all cases. Among the adult cases, the causes of death were intracerebral hemorrhage in 33 cases (including 26 of ventricular rupture), intraventricular hemorrhage in 7 cases, subdural hematoma in 1 case, and subarachnoid hemorrhage in 1 case. There was a high incidence of ventricular hemorrhage. Cerebral infarction was the cause of death in only six cases. Among juvenile cases, on the other hand, there was one case of intracerebral hemorrhage, one case of subdural hematoma, one case of aneurysm rupture, and two cases of infectious disease. The fact that the immediate cause of death was cerebral angiography itself in three cases clearly indicates the need for sufficient care in performing angiography in cases of moyamoya disease, which is essentially a form of obstructive cerebrovascular disease.

The course from onset until death is known in 30 cases. Among the juvenile cases, the entire course ran 6 months at the most rapid and 7 years at the slowest. Among adult cases, the entire course ran a matter of 2 days in the fastest case, whereas in the slowest case onset was in childhood and death due to cerebral hemorrhage did not occur until 17 years later.

10.3 Pathology of Autopsied Brain Tissue

The macroscopic findings of autopsied brain depended largely on the clinical course of the disease and the actual cause of death. As summarized in Fig. 99, there were cases in which intracerebral hemorrhage and its rupture into the ventricles were seen, cases in which there was only subarachnoid hemorrhage or ventricular hemorrhage, case with limited infarctic lesions, cases with diffuse and marked infarctic lesions, cases of cerebral atrophy, cases with both hemorrhagic and infarctic lesions, etc. This diversity of brain lesions was naturally enough reflected in a similar diversity of clinical features.

Study of the cut surface of the brain showed anastomosis of tortuous perforators in the cerebrum (Fig. 100) [2, 16, 23, 61, 76, 78, 81, 102, 122, 167, 168, 226, 229, 231, 339] and there were groups of dilatated small vessels on the brain surface [5, 16, 102, 122, 229], particularly at the base of the frontal lobe and in the vicinity of the olfactory nerves (Fig. 101).

10.3.1 Pathology of the Foci of Cerebral Hemorrhage

Among the 44 cases of death by hemorrhage, 35 were cases of intracerebral hermorrhage. Of these, 28 had ventricular rupture, with 7 having primary intraventricular hemorrhage, a rather high incidence of intraventricular hemorrhage. According to Tanaka et al. [227, 322, 323], although there are some cases in which the intracerebral hermorrhage ruptures the cerebral cortex and emerges at the surface of the brain, most cases show hermorrhage at the basal ganglia, thalamus, or hypothalamus which ruptures into the cerebral ventricles.

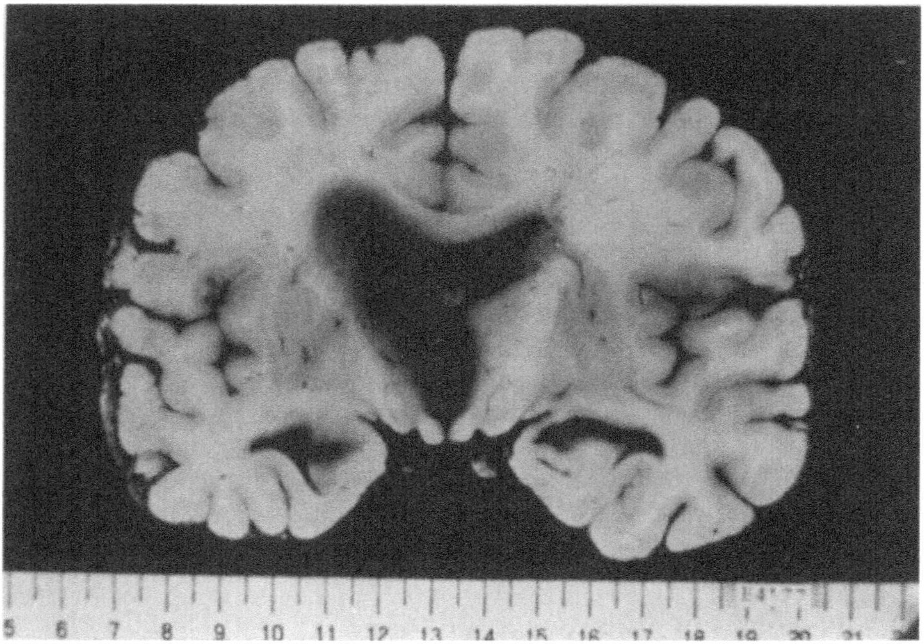

Fig. 99. Right thalamic hemorrhage rupture to the ventricle, filling the ventricular system, and subarachnoid hemorrhage on the brain surface

The identification of ruptured vessels is a difficult problem in moyamoya disease. We have previously reported on the possibility of hemorrhage from moyamoya vessels of the superior lateral region of the body of the lateral ventricle due to vascular weakening caused by chronic ischemia or a mechanism similar to hemorrhagic infarction of an infarctic lesion [133]. In general, however, it is thought that hemorrhage most frequently occurs from moyamoya vessels (anastomatic channels) which are intracerebral near the ventricles or in the ventricular walls [37, 86, 172, 224, 270, 322, 323].

Various facts point to the likelihood of hemorrhage in this region. The walls of moyamoya vessels are only 10 μm thick, suggesting that rupture could easily occur [37]. Pathological changes are seen similar to the moth-eaten appearance of the tunica media seen in the peripheral perforators in hypertensive disorders, and these suggest the possibility of direct arterial rupture without the development of angionecrosis or other pathological changes [172]. Moreover, the vessels in the hemorrhagic focus and the immediate periphery show clear disruption of the wall structure and the typical precursor pathology of arterial necrosis by plasma. Such findings suggest the presence of extremely abnormal local hemodynamics. These changes found in moyamoya disease are thought likely to develop into microaneurysms or arterial necrosis.

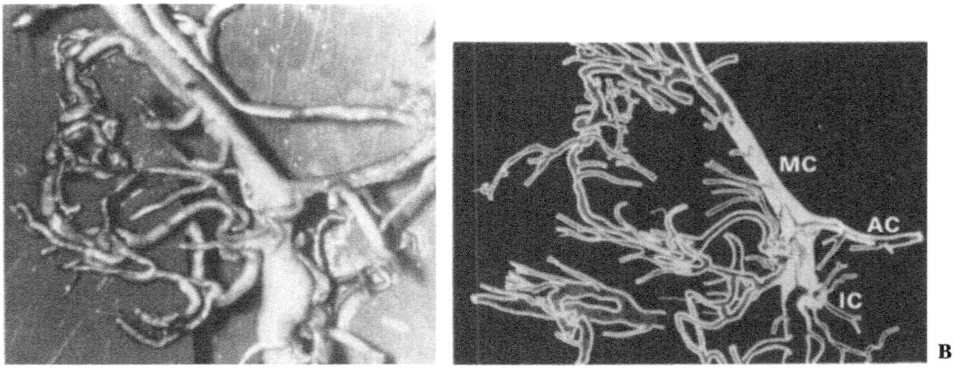

A B

Fig. 100 A, B. Main cerebral arteries and perforating branches of an autopsied brain. Remarkable stenotic change of the carotid fork and anastomoses between the perforating branches are seen. **A** Specimen of the carotid fork. **B** Schema of **A** (showing thickness of walls and lumens). *MC*, middle cerebral artery; *AC*, anterior cerebral artery; *IC*, internal carotid artery

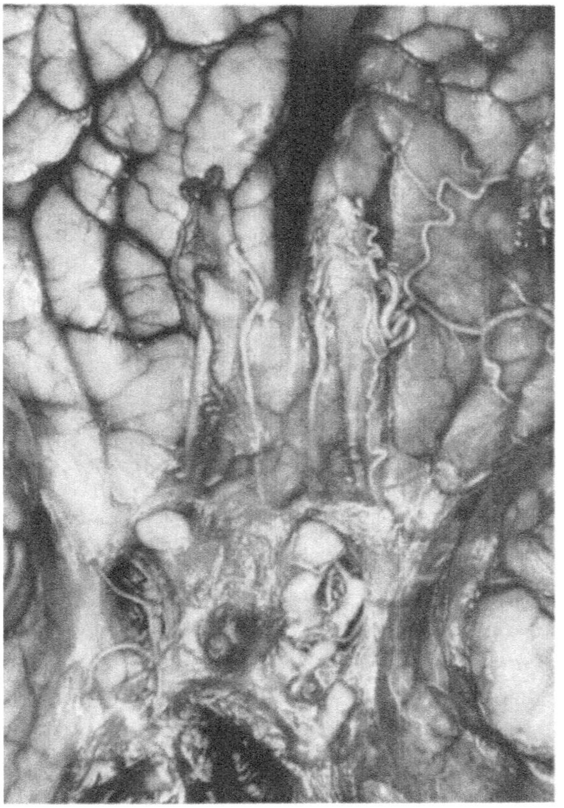

Fig. 101. The base of the frontal lobe of an autopsied brain. Many dilated and tortuous small arteries are observed in the vicinity of the olfactory bulbs

10.3.2 Pathology of Infarctic Foci

Infarction is often found in moyamoya disease, but death due to cerebral infarction is uncommon [323]. Infarctic foci have been classified into two separate groups [321] : (a) those which are found diffusely or as multiple lesions in the cortex and white matter in the region supplied by the anterior and middle cerebral arteries and (b) those that are found in the region supplied by the perforating branches in the vicinity of the walls of the lateral and third ventricles.

It is not always the case that the location of the infarctic focus coincides with that of the stenotic changes in the feeding arteries, but it is widely held that the development of collateral pathways plays a role in limiting the extent of cerebral infarction [224, 321]. There are also cases in which thrombus formation is seen, and such thrombi are thought to be involved not only in the development of arterial pathology, but also in the development of brain ischemia [86, 321, 323]. Particularly the thrombi seen in the lenticulostriate artery and in the thalamoperforate artery are thought to play an important role in the development of brain infarction [320].

10.3.3 Pathology of the Trunk Arteries at the Base of the Brain

The fundamental architecture of the circle of Willis is well developed in both juvenile and adult cases of moyamoya disease, but there is vascular narrowing due to stenotic and obstructive changes in the main trunk arteries of the brain, i. e., the terminal portion of the internal carotid artery and the origins of the anterior cerebral artery and the middle cerebral artery. In general, there are few changes in the posterior communicating artery, the posterior cerebral artery, and the vertebrobasilar system, although dilatation of these vessels is sometimes found [193] (Fig. 98).

Such stenosis and obstruction of the trunk arteries around the carotid fork bilaterally are due to fibrous or cellular-fibrous thickening of the intima in both juvenile and adult cases [193, 298], and layered structures due to elastic fiber growth are also seen. The internal elastic lamina shows tortuosity and duplication, whereas the media shows atrophy and thinning. The adventitia does not normally show marked changes (Figs. 102, 103). In general, these vessels do not show arteriosclerotic or inflammatory changes, such as cell infiltration [23, 61, 71, 78, 231, 256, 298, 339]. The above changes are the typical pathological findings in moyamoya disease, but there are considerable individual differences in the location, severity, and qualitative nature of these changes.

Among the qualitative differences that can be found, there is calcification [5, 6, 78], hyaline degeneration [167, 168], and cholesterine deposits of the intima [225], recanalization of platelet thrombi [22, 83, 120], and infiltration of round cells into the adventitia [76, 167, 168]. Among differences in severity, there are various degrees of intimal thickening, ranging from no stenosis to complete occlusion. Among variations in location, there are even cases of medial thickening

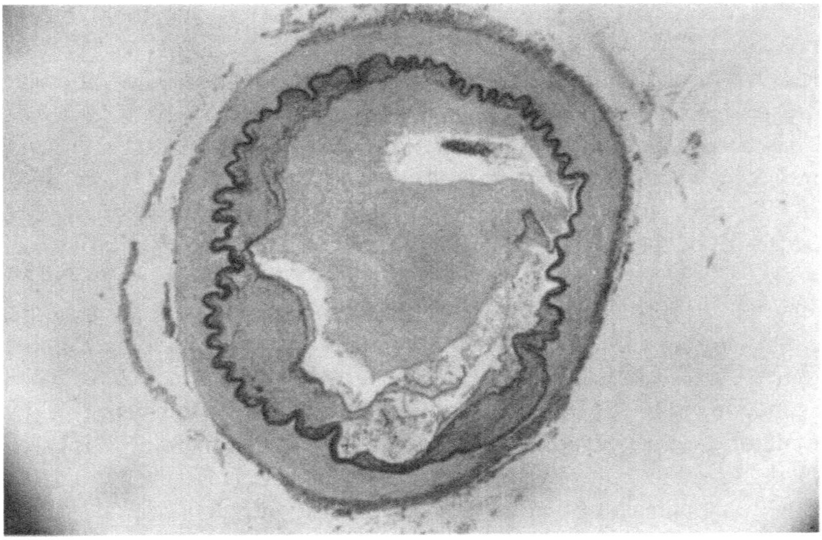

Fig. 102. Microsection of left internal carotid artery (C_1). Elastica-Masson stain, x 40. An eccentric narrowing of the lumen — due to a cellular-fibrous thickening of the intima, a tortuosity, and a duplication of the internal elastic lamina — and a thinning of the media due to atrophy are observed

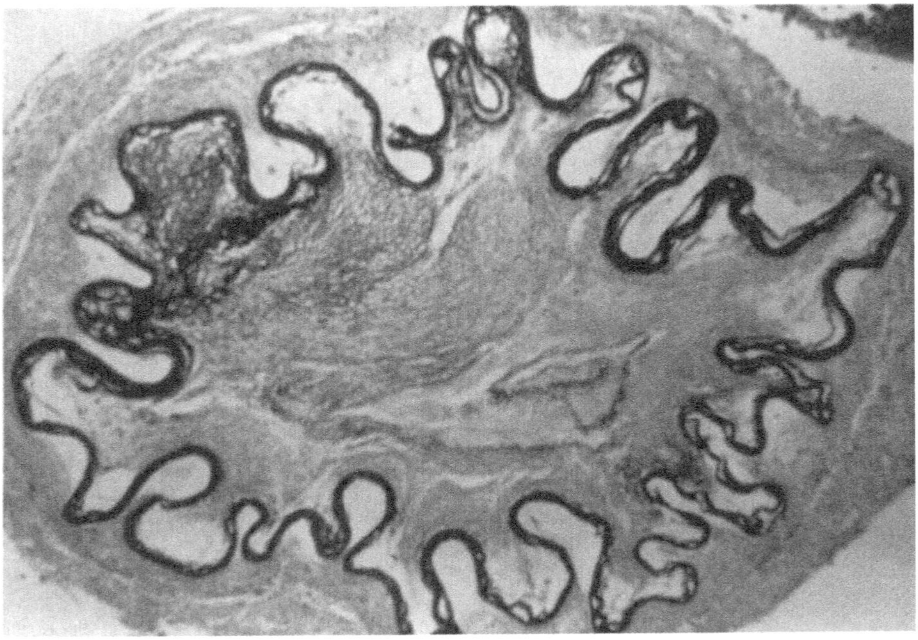

Fig. 103. Microsection of the A_1 portion of the right anterior cerebral artery, showing a cellular-fibrous thickening of the intima, a tortuosity, a duplication of the internal elastic lamina, and a marked thinning of the media x 100

of the posterior communicating artery and the vertebrobasilar artery [61, 226, 320] (Fig. 104).

Among adult cases of moyamoya disease, however, there are cases showing arteriosclerosis as well as ones showing calcification [5, 6, 78], atheroma [172, 270, 320], and atheroma together with hyalinization of the intima [229]. Moreover, there are also cases with infiltration of round cells into the adventitia [76, 167, 168], infiltration of lymphocytes into the media or adventitia [102], and thickening [229, 339] or fibrosis [6] of the adventitia. These aspects differ from the pathology in juvenile cases.

With regard to the obstructive findings of the trunk arteries near the terminal portion of the internal carotid artery both congenital and acquired factors are thought to be involved. Principal among the hypotheses which have been suggested concerning the etiology of moyamoya disease are the following:

1. The vascular hypoplasia hypothesis [2, 102, 122, 270]. This hypothesis is based upon the argument that moyamoya disease may develop due to the hypoplastic arteries with hypoplasia of the media and tortuosity and local defects of the internal elastic lamina.
2. The polster hypothesis [16, 22, 61]. In this hypothesis, it is maintained that vascular stenosis is due to the abnormal proliferation of polsters during fetal development, their subsequent spread and, moreover, platelet thrombus formation.

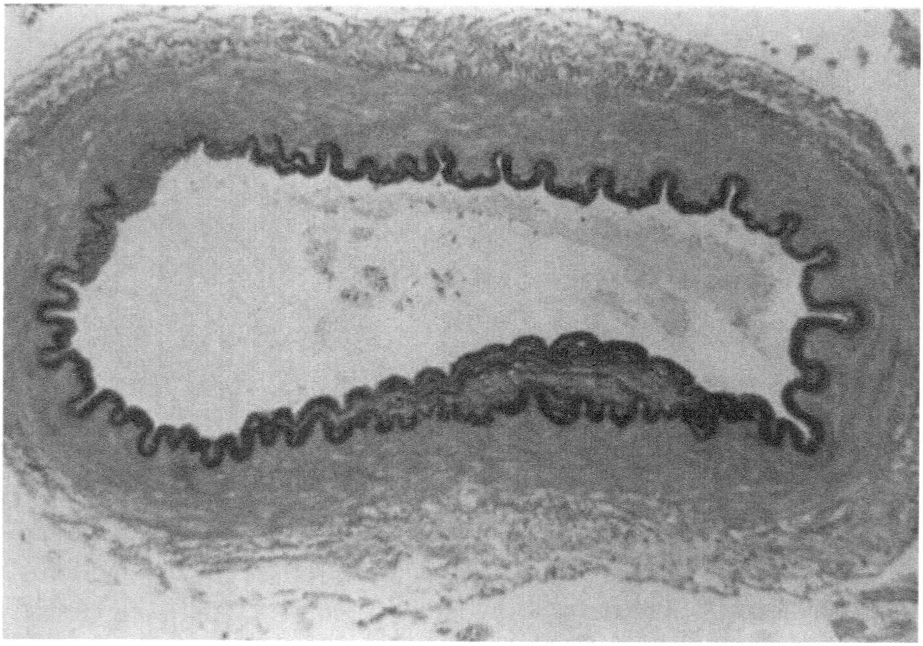

Fig. 104. Microsection of the left posterior communicating artery, showing a thickened media and partial elastosis x 100

3. The remnant fetal vascular network hypothesis [165, 213].
4. The angiomatous malformation around the terminal portion of the internal carotid artery hypothesis [153, 167].
5. The stenosis due to thrombus formation in the internal carotid artery hypothesis [37].
6. The arteriosclerotic change hypothesis [56, 76, 78, 82–84, 225, 229]. In this hypothesis, it is maintained that the original cause is juvenile intimal arteriosclerosis with its characteristic diffuse thickening of the intima [56, 76, 78, 84]. Abnormalities of vascular permeability and the involvement of serum components in the vascular wall [164, 170, 225] are originally induced, followed by white thrombus formation in the vascular walls and their organization [229] – eventually leading to vascular obstruction.
7. The inflammation hypothesis. In this hypothesis it is maintained that infection is involved [120] and vascular occlusion is a direct result of arteritis [6, 95]. Contrarily, it has been suggested that the gradual and repeated inflammation of the head and neck causes an immune reaction mediated through the superior cervical ganglions which spreads to the bifurcation of the internal carotid artery [115, 137, 299].
8. The cerebral vasospasm hypothesis [172].

10.3.4 Pathology of the Moyamoya Vessels

It is well known that in both juvenile and adult moyamoya disease there is abnormal development of the perforating branches of thin arteries within the basal cistern, centering around the circle of Willis. Depending upon the individual case, moyamoya vessels are found primarily in the vicinity of the internal carotid artery, anterior choroidal artery, middle cerebral artery, anterior cerebral artery, or posterior communicating artery. These moyamoya vessels are found to have dilatated and to have formed vascular nets through anastomosis (Fig. 100) and to have had communication with cortical branches (Fig. 105). Such marked development of these vascular nets is not restricted to the basal cisterns, but can be found in the leptomeninges of the brain surface [5, 59, 81, 120, 167, 225, 226, 256, 339] and dilatated vessels can also be seen on the cut surface of the brain (Fig. 100) [5, 23, 59, 100, 120, 175, 270].

Moyamoya vessels are known to be dilatated arterial vessels with thin walls and complicated configuration, but it is thought that thickening of the intima and elastosis do not occur [16, 56, 61, 76, 122, 231]. However, the walls of such dilatated vessels are thin, the internal elastic lamina is not distinct, and they appear either much like venous vessels or it is unclear whether they are arterial or venous in origin [56, 61, 225, 226] (Fig. 106). There have also been reports of vessels with hypertrophy of the muscle cells of the media [78, 229, 297]. Among adult cases, however, there have been cases of obstruction due to severe fibroelastosis [61, 102, 165, 172, 231, 321–323] and, among cases of obstruction, there have also been reports of organized thrombi [226, 322].

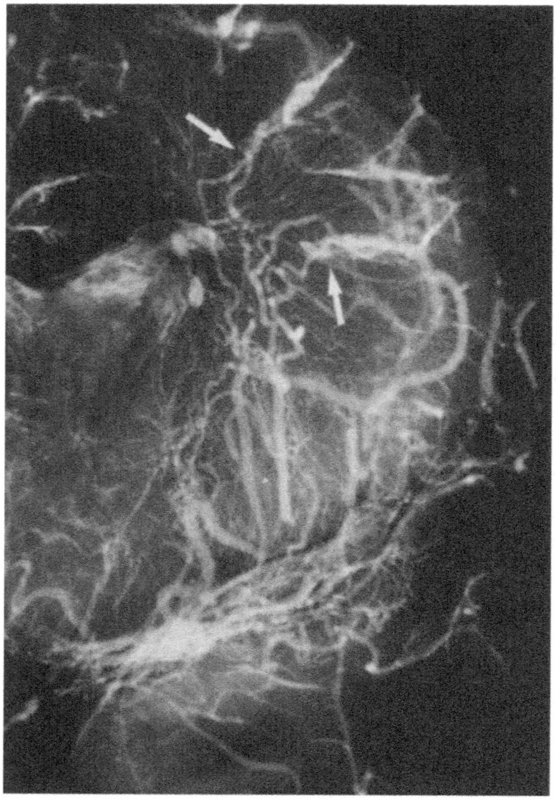

Fig. 105. Microangiogram of an adult autopsied brain. Communications between moyamoya vessels at the basal ganglia and cortical branches of the middle cerebral artery (*arrow*) are observed

10.4 Investigations Based upon Whole Body Autopsy

A total of 32 whole body autopsy cases of moyamoya disease, including three of our own [193, 298], have been reported in the literature. These include 7 juvenile cases (ages 2–16 years), 16 adult cases (ages 24–66 years), and 9 cases reported by Tanaka [323], whose ages were not clearly stated [2, 5, 6, 22, 23, 37, 59, 76, 78, 120, 165, 175, 225, 226, 229, 231, 270, 339].

In all but one juvenile case [22] and three adult cases [6, 270, 339], several abnormal changes in arterial vessels were found at locations in the body other than the brain. In both juvenile and adult cases, vascular changes similar to those found in the cerebral vessels were seen, including sclerotic changes in the aorta and coronary artery and intimal hypertrophy of the coronary, renal, and pulmonary arteries (Fig. 107).

Hosoda and Ishii [84] have reported severe atheromatous sclerosis of the terminal portion of the internal carotid artery in a 24-year-old female case of moyamoya disease. They also found sclerosis of the coronary and renal arteries.

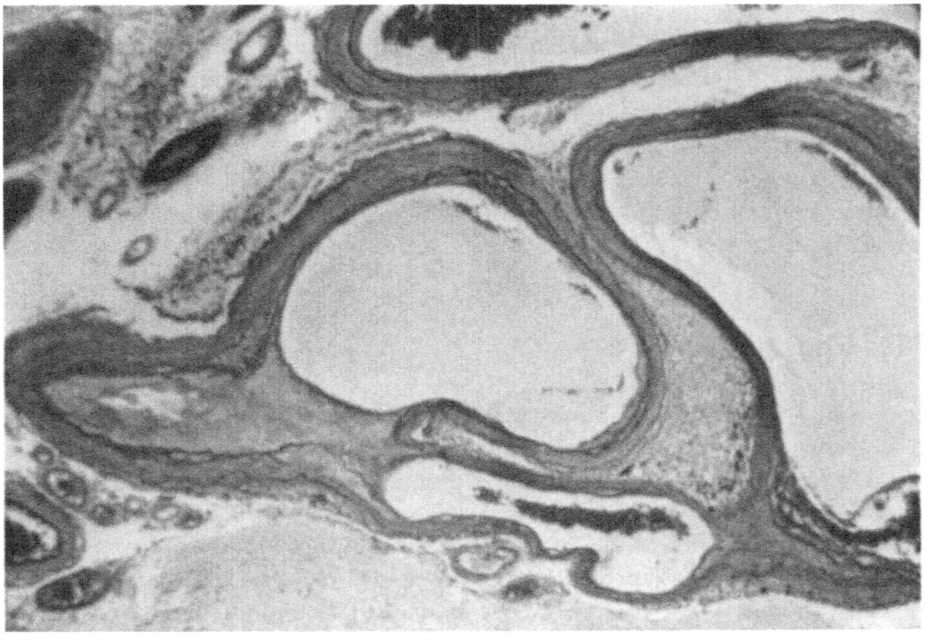

Fig. 106. Microsection of moyamoya vessels, showing vascular findings with dilated lumens and thinned walls. It is unclear whether they are arterial or venous in origin. Hematoxylin-eosin stain, x 200

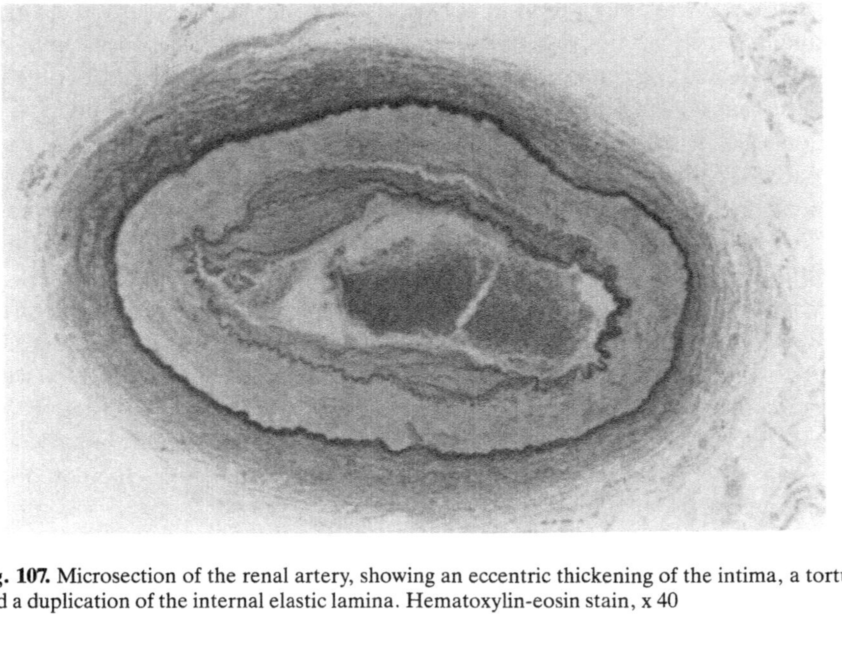

Fig. 107. Microsection of the renal artery, showing an eccentric thickening of the intima, a tortuosity, and a duplication of the internal elastic lamina. Hematoxylin-eosin stain, x 40

From the fact that lipid deposits (which were severe considering the age of the patient) were seen on the aorta, Hosoda maintains that a clear distinction between the pathology described above and that of normally progressing arteriosclerosis can be made. He advocates the term »juvenile arteriosclerosis« for such pathology. In other words, moyamoya disease in this view may be a »partial« or »cerebral« type of systemic arterial pathology [193, 299]. If this is the case, then moyamoya disease should be understood and investigated in relation to the entire arterial vascular system [35, 66].

10.5 Conclusion

In moyamoya disease, the greatest remaining problems concern its pathogenesis. It is known that the pathology of moyamoya disease involves the progressive stenosis and obstruction of the bilateral terminal portions of the internal carotid artery. Histopathologically, the basic and common changes include eccentric and laminated hypertrophy of the intima, abnormal tortuosity and duplication of the internal elastic lamina, and thinning of the media. Because some changes other than those described above were seen due to differences in other factors contributing to the pathogenesis in individual cases, various interpretations have been made concerning the fundamental pathology. Consequently, it would appear that elucidation of the essential nature of moyamoya disease solely from a pathological viewpoint remains difficult.

It is known that changes in arterial walls can be brought about by various factors, ultimately resulting in intimal hypertrophy and arteriosclerotic changes. Consequently, the pathology seen in autopsy cases of moyamoya desease may not provide conclusive answers concerning its pathogenesis, as suggested by Angeline [6]: »These findings are interpreted as a late stage of the disease and give no indications as to its pathogenesis.« Of course, it can easily be suggested that study of the pathology of moyamoya disease in the chronic, subacute, and acute stages might lead to the elucidation of the pathognomonic characteristics unique to moyamoya disease, but, practically speaking, it is exceedingly difficult to examine pathologically all the stages of the disease.

It remains difficult to generalize on the pathology of moyamoya disease on the basis of any single autopsy study, and each individual case must be considered in relation to the pathology arising at various stages in the disease. Only when autopsy studies are made prospectively with a consistent perspective will generalizations become possible. Currently, it must be concluded that research solely from the vantage point of autopsy studies has not elucidated the fundamental pathology of moyamoya disease.

11 Etiology

11.1 Introduction

Twenty years have passed since attention was drawn to moyamoya disease as a distinct disease entity, but as yet no theory has become established concerning the direct cause of the stenotic changes in the terminal portion of the internal carotid artery, which are thought to be the earliest pathological changes in this disease [61, 78, 81, 142, 167, 184, 213, 258, 289, 313]. In recent years, the participation of HLA antigens [124] and autologous antibodies in moyamoya disease has been suggested, but no hypothesis has yet found direct empirical support and, in fact, there has been virtually no experimental research [311] on its etiology.

Consequently, we have undertaken an experimental study on the cause of the stenotic changes near the terminal portion of the internal carotid artery using a canine model. Here the results of this study are reported we discuss our current thoughts on the etiology of moyamoya disease [115, 354].

11.2 Background to Our Experimental Research

As discussed in previous chapters, pathological findings on the main cerebral arteries, particularly at the carotid fork, in moyamoya disease include cellular and fibrous thickening of the intima, tortuosity, rupturing and duplication of the internal elastic lamina, and thinning of the tunica media (Figs. 102, 105). These findings are similar to the pathological findings for chronic lesions of vasculitis [127], thought to be due to an immune reaction, such as found in polyarteritis [187, 359] and Kawasaki's disease [10, 324].

In the previous chapter, it was mentioned that similar pathological change is found in the arteries of organs other than the brain with a high frequency in autopsy studies of moyamoya disease cases. It is therefore thought that moyamoya disease may be a form of generalized vasculitis in which the pathological change is particularly advanced in the cerebral arteries. On the other hand, it is also known that patients with moyamoya disease frequently have a history of reccurent and chronic infections above the neck, particularly tonsillitis. There have also been a large number of cases in which a fever of unknown cause arose immediately prior to onset of moyamoya disease as well as a larger number of cases in which some form of precursor infection has been suggested. These facts suggest that during the recovery from the transient appearance of a specific, relatively mild form of vasculitis, or due to the repeated occurrence of such a process, the above-mentioned vascular pathology may eventually emerge.

11.3 Experimental Methods and Results

In the first part of this experimental study, three dogs were used (Nos. 1–3) (Tables 19, 20). Systemic sensitization was undertaken with heterologous serum in order to produce vasculitis due to serum sickness. Vascular changes were found in all three animals, although one showed only unilateral changes. Significantly, the vascular changes were confined to the main arteries at the base of the brain, centering around the terminal portion of the carotid artery. No such pathology

Table 19. Experimental methods and results

Dog No.	Sex	SCG	Antigen	GS	LS	Last GS or LS before killed	Arterial changes: Cerebral artery		Renal artery
1	♂	(+)	Cat S	SC x 4	–	3 days	R(+)	L(+)	(+)
2	♀	(+)	Cat S	SC x 8, IV x 2	–	1 day	R(+)	L(+)	(–)
3	♀	(+)	Cat S	SC x 10, IV x 5	–	1 day	R(–)	L(+)	(–)
4	♂	(+)	Cat S	SC x 2	R LN x 6	1 day	R(+)	L(+)	(–)
5	♀	(+)	Cat S	SC x 2	R LN x 4	1 day	R(+)	L(+)	(–)
6	♂	(+)	Cat S	SC x 2	R LN x 5	1 month	R(–)	L(–)	(–)
7	♂	(+)	Cat S	SC x 5	R SCG x 3	1 day	R(+)	L(–)	(+)
8	♀	(+)	Cat S	SC x 4	R SCG x 2	1 day	R(+)	L(–)	(–)
9	♀	(+)	Horse S	SC x 9	R SCG x 11	1 day	R(+)	L(+)	(+)
10	♂	(+)	Cat S	SC x 9	R SCG x 7	7 h	R(+)	L(+)	(–)
11	♀	(+)	Horse S	SC x 9	R SCG x 9	1 day	R(+)	L(+)	(–)
12	♂	(+)	Cat S	SC x 4	R SCG x 4	8 days	R(–)	L(–)	(–)
13	♀	(+)	Cat S	SC x 7	R·L SCG x 5	1 day	R(+)	L(+)	(+)
14	♀	(+)	Cat S	SC x 7	R·L SCG x 5	1 day	R(+)	L(+)	(–)
15	♀	(+)	Cat S	SC x 6	R·L SCG x 4	1 day	R(+)	L(+)	(–)
16	♂	R(–) L(+)	Horse S	SC x 5, IV x 3	L SCG x 3	1 day	R(–)	L(+)	(+)
17	♀	R(–) L(+)	Cat S	SC x 8	L SCG x 6	1 day	R(–)	L(+)	(–)
18	♀	R(–) L(+)	Horse S	SC x 7	L SCG x 5	1 day	R(+)	L(+)	(+)
19	♂	R(–) L(+)	Cat S	SC x 6, IV x 9	L SCG x 6	3 h	R(–)	L(+)	(–)
20	♂	R(–) L(+)	Cat S	SC x 8, IV x 8	L SCG x 6	3 h	R(–)	L(+)	(+)
21	♀	R(–) L(+)	Cat S	SC x 8, IV x 11	L SCG x 5	3 h	R(+)	L(+)	(+)
22	♂	R(–) L(+)	β-Str	L SCG (abscess)	β-Str x 5	1 day	R(+)	L(+)	(–)
23	♂	R(–) L(+)	β-Str	L SCG (abscess)	β-Str x 31	1 day	R(–)	L(+)	(–)
24	♂	R(–) L(+)	β-Str	L SCG (abscess)	β-Str x 21	1 day	R(+)	L(+)	(+)
25	♀	(+)	(–)	(–)	(–)		R(–)	L(–)	(–)
26	♂	(+)	(–)	(–)	(–)		R(–)	L(–)	(–)

SCG, superior cervical ganglion; GS, general sensitization; LS, local stimulation; LN, lymph node; SC, subcutaneous injection; IV, intravenous injection; β-Str, β-Streptococcus hemolyticus; R, right; L, left; R·L, right and left; S, serum

Table 20. Location and degree of cerebral arterial changes in general sensitization

No.		CIC	IC	M_1	A_1	PCOM	PC	$M_{2\text{-}5}$	$A_{2\text{-}5}$	BA
1	R	(+)	(⧻)	(−)	(−)	(−)	(−)	(−)	(−)	(−)
	L	(⧺)	(−)	(−)	(⧺)	(−)	(−)	(−)	(−)	(−)
2	R	(+)	(−)	(−)	(−)	(−)	(−)	(−)	(−)	(−)
	L	(+)	(−)	(−)	(−)	(−)	(−)	(−)	(−)	(−)
3	R	(−)	(−)	(−)	(−)	(−)	(−)	(−)	(−)	(−)
	L	(+)	(−)	(−)	(−)	(−)	(−)	(−)	(−)	(−)

CIC, cavernous portion of internal carotid artery; IC, intracranial internal carotid artery; M_1, M_1 portion of middle cerebral artery; A_1, A_1 portion of anterior cerebral artery; PCOM, posterior communicating artery; PC, posterior cerebral artery; $M_{2\text{-}5}$, $M_{2\text{-}5}$ portions of middle cerebral artery; $A_{s\text{-}5}$, $A_{2\text{-}5}$, portions of anterior cerebral artery; BA, basilar artery; (+), change of one layer out of intimal thickening, elastosis, and myonecrosis; (⧺), changes of two layers; (⧻), changes of three layers

was found on the basilar artery or on peripheral arteries. The vascular changes were all mild, but included eccentric proliferation of the intima (Figs. 108, 110), tortuosity, rupture and duplication of the internal elastic lamina (Figs. 109, 110), and myonecrosis of the tunica media (Fig. 111). Moreover, thrombus formation was occasionally seen at the site of rupture of the intima and the internal elastic lamina (Fig. 109). These findings were suggestive of the early-stage vascular changes found in moyamoya disease. The pathological changes in the vessels were found from the intima through the muscular layers of the media, with no changes in the adventitia.

Cochrane et al. [25, 30, 155, 156] originally proposed that the vascular changes caused by an immune reaction are due to immune complexes in the blood entering the vascular walls, which have increased permeability. It was therefore of great interest that the vascular changes seen in our experimental preparations were also found to occur from the intimal side and extending toward, but not including, the adventitia. In order to test whether or not such changes were due to an immune mechanism, the following experiment [353] was undertaken.

Four dogs were prepared using the same procedure as described above for producing vascular changes, and sequential measurements were made of the antibody titers following sensitization to antigen. Sharp increases in antibody titers were seen in all four dogs about 5 days following the first general, subcutaneous sensitization procedure. By subsequently injecting antigen intravenously in three dogs, sharp decreases in antibody titer were then found in all three (Fig. 112). This finding is thought to indicate that the large volume of antigen injected intravenously formed immune complexes with the antibody already present in the bloodstream. Free antibody would then be consumed in the process of complex formation, and the volume of free antibody greatly reduced. In other words, this experiment gaves indirect confirmation of the occurrence of an immune reaction.

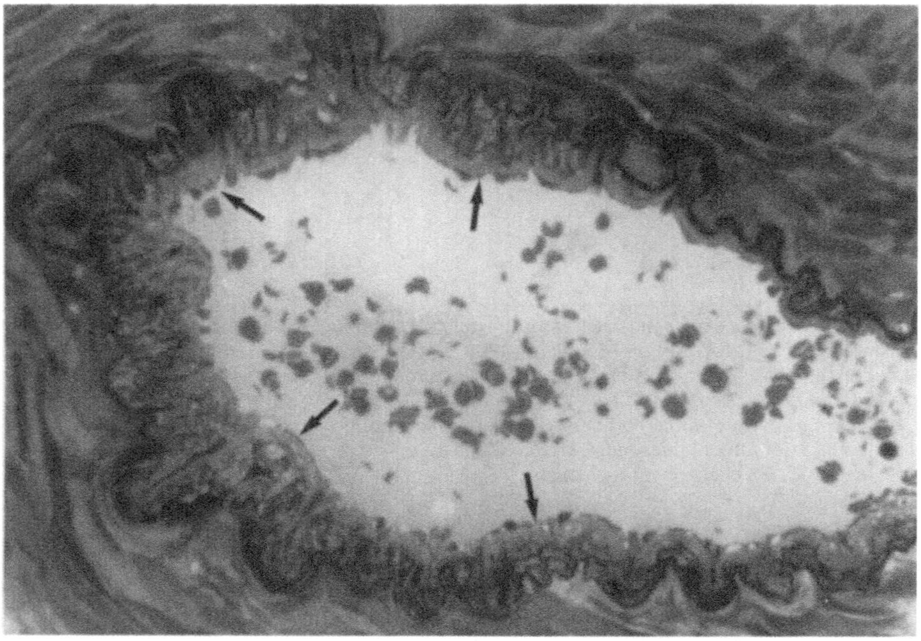

Fig. 108. Microsection of the terminal portion of the intracranial internal carotid artery showing eccentric proliferation of the intima (*arrows*) (Dog No. 7). Toluidine blue stain, x 200

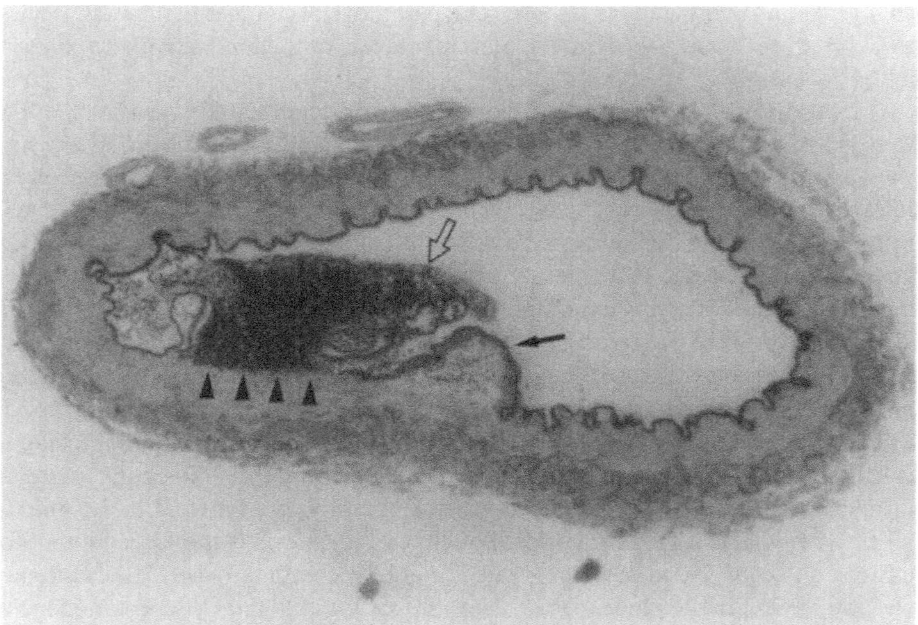

Fig. 109. Microsection of the terminal portion of the intracranial internal carotid artery showing destruction (▶) and tortuosity (➧) of internal elastic lamina associated with thrombus formation (⇨) (Dog No. 16). (Elastica-Masson stain, x 40)

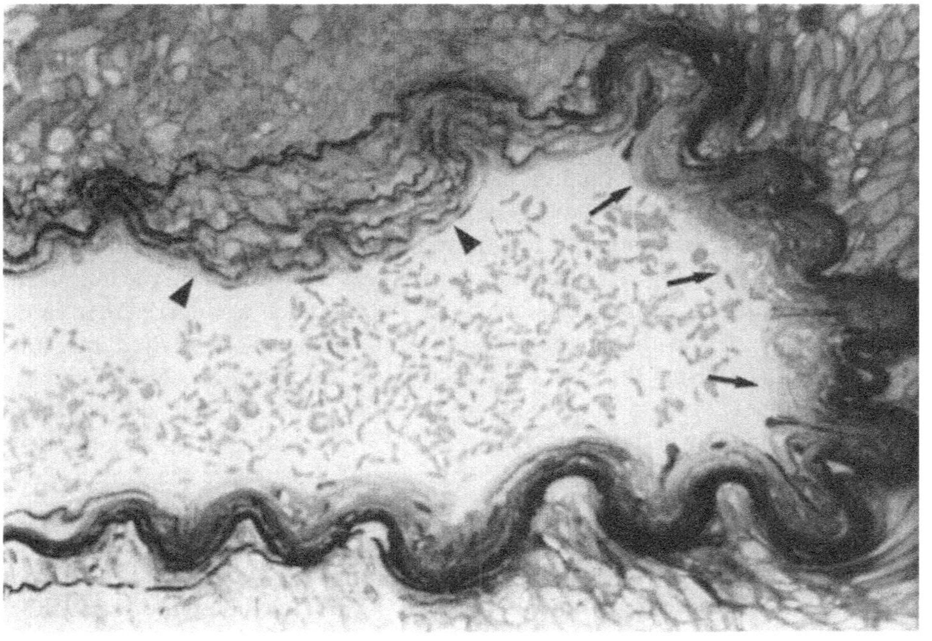

Fig. 110. Microsection of the terminal portion of the intracranial internal carotid artery showing partial elastosis (▶) and eccentric proliferation of the intima (➧) (Dog No. 1). Toluidine blue stain, x 200

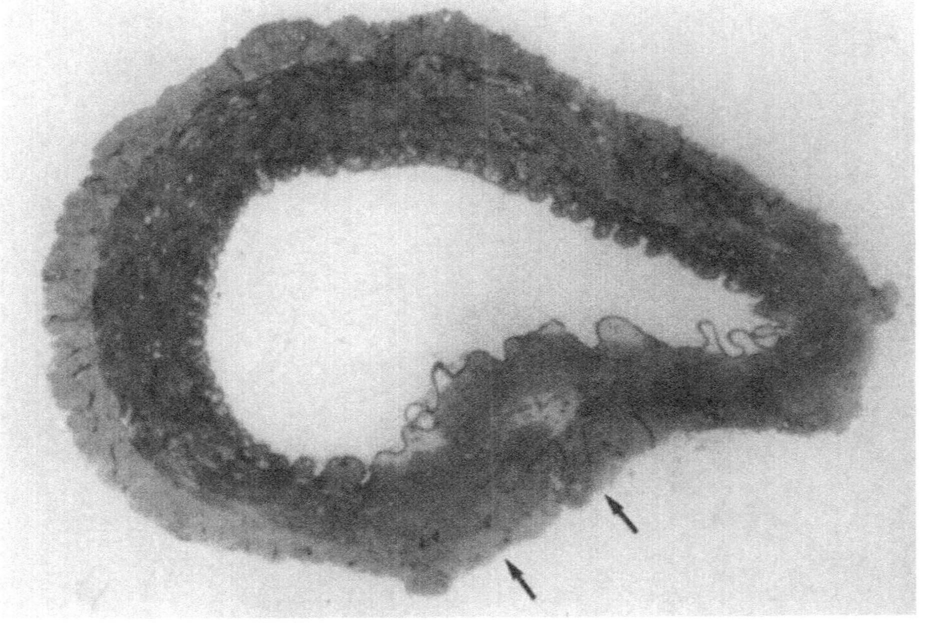

Fig. 111. Microsection of the terminal portion of the intracranial internal carotid artery showing partial myonecrosis (➧) and tortuosity of internal elastic lamina (Dog No. 1). Toluidine blue stain, x 40

In the main arteries at the base of the brain in the dogs killed at the end of the experiments, there were destructive changes in blood vessels, primarily in the intima and in the internal elastic lamina. There was also intimal thickening which was thought to be due to so-called »endarteritis« and its repair.

We next undertook an immunohistological investigation of the presence and distribution of antigen, antibody, and complement in the trunk arteries at the base of the brain. First, an immunoflorescent study of antigen in the vascular walls was made. It was found (Fig. 113) that antigen was present primarily in the intima and directly beneath the internal elastic lamina, with antigen sometimes seen in the media. Study of the distribution of IgG and IgM antibodies and the third complement (C_3) using the same method showed the antibodies distributed in a manner similar to antigen, i. e., in the intima, directly beneath the internal elastic lamina, and sparsely in the media (Figs. 114, 115). In contrast, C_3 was confined to the intima and there was considerably less complement there than antibody or antigen (Fig. 116).

Using an enzyme-antibody technique, findings identical to those obtained with the fluorescent method were obtained concerning both antigen and antibody (Fig. 117). From these immunological results, it was concluded that the vascular changes found in these dogs were due to an immune reaction.

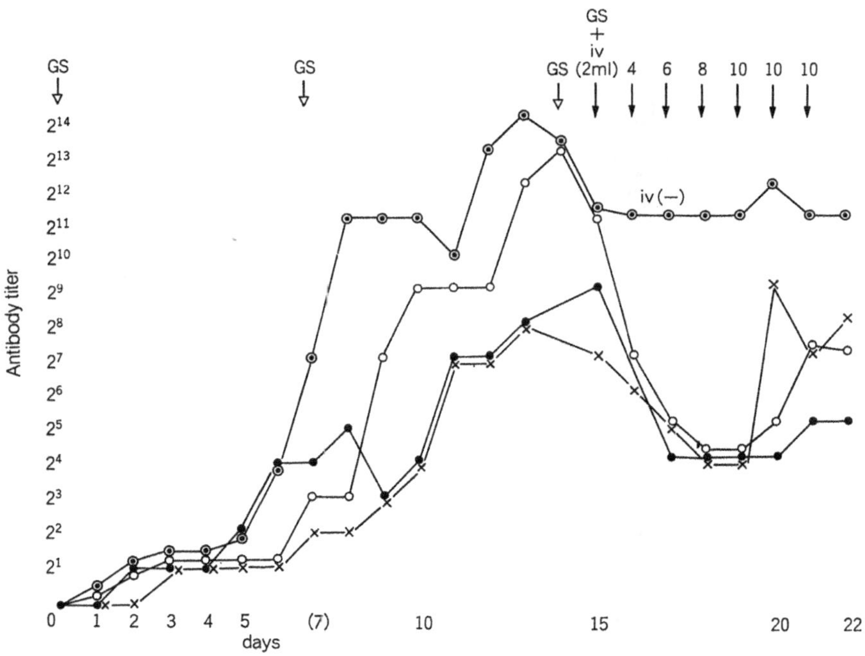

Fig. 112. Sequential changes of the antibody titers in blood of experimental dogs. *GS*, general sensitization by subcutaneous injections of heterologous serum. *iv*, general sensitization by intravenous injections of heterologous serum

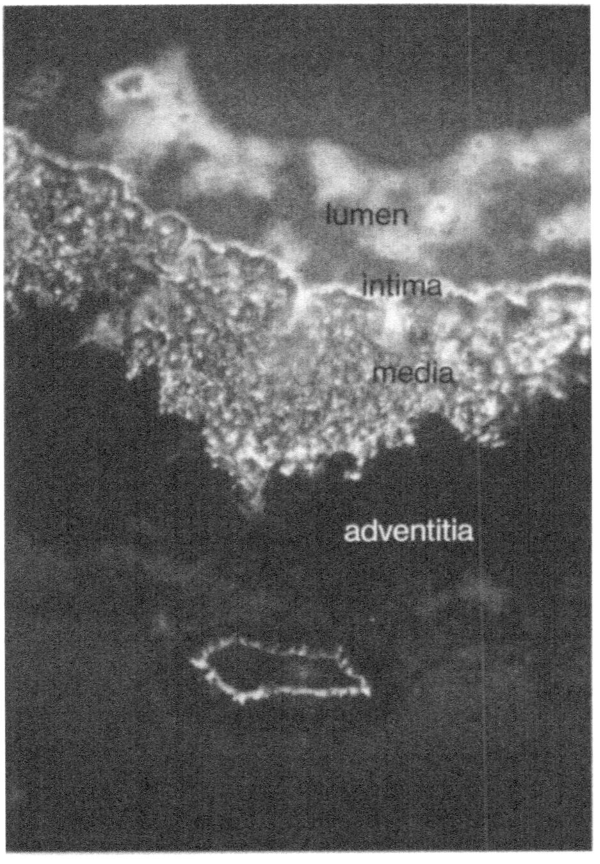

Fig. 113. Investigation of the antigen by an immunofluorescent study. Antibodies are diffusely present from the intima to the media (the terminal portion of the intracranial internal carotid artery). x 200

It is of considerable interest that the distribution of antibody and antigen in the cerebral vessels of three dogs (Nos. 22–24) was particularly dense at the anterior portion of the circle of Willis, including all of the perforating branches at the base of the brain. In contrast, no such vascular change was found on the vertebral or basilar arteries. This pattern of vascular change correlates closely with that seen in moyamoya disease (Table 21).

As mentioned earlier, the vascular pathology in moyamoya disease is found primarily on the anterior half of the circle of Willis, centering on the terminal portion of the internal carotid artery. In immunological vasculitis, such as in aortitis syndrome and polyarteritis, there are also sites in the vascular system which are particularly susceptible. The causes of the localized vascular changes in both immunological vasculitis and moyamoya disease, however, have remained uncertain. And this question concerning the factors behind the localization of disease has motivated the present experiments.

Table 21. Distribution of the antigen and the antibody in the main arteries at the base of the brain in experimental dogs. Localized sites of existence of the antigen and the antibody were proved in the main arteries at the anterior half of the circle of Willis, centering on the terminal portion of the internal carotid artery, where vascular changes occurred correspondingly

No.		CIC	IC	M_1	A_1	PCOM	PC	BA
22	R	(+)	(+)	(+)	(−)	(+)	(−)	(−)
	L	(+)	(+)	(+)	(−)	(−)	(−)	
23	R	(−)	(+)	(+)	(+)	(−)	(−)	(−)
	L	(+)	(+)	(+)	(−)	(−)	(−)	
24	R	(+)	(+)	(+)	(+)	(+)		(−)
	L	(+)	(+)	(+)	(+)	(+)	(−)	

Abbreviations as for Table 20

Based on the fact that the sites at which the early vascular changes in moyamoya disease coincided with the sites of vascular pathology in our animal experiments and the sites where antigen, antibody, and complement were most abundantly located, i.e., at the terminal portion of the internal carotid artery, further efforts were made to elucidate what the determining factor in the vascular pathology is. First, it was considered that a solely immunological explanation of the localization of the vascular changes would not suffice. That is, there must be

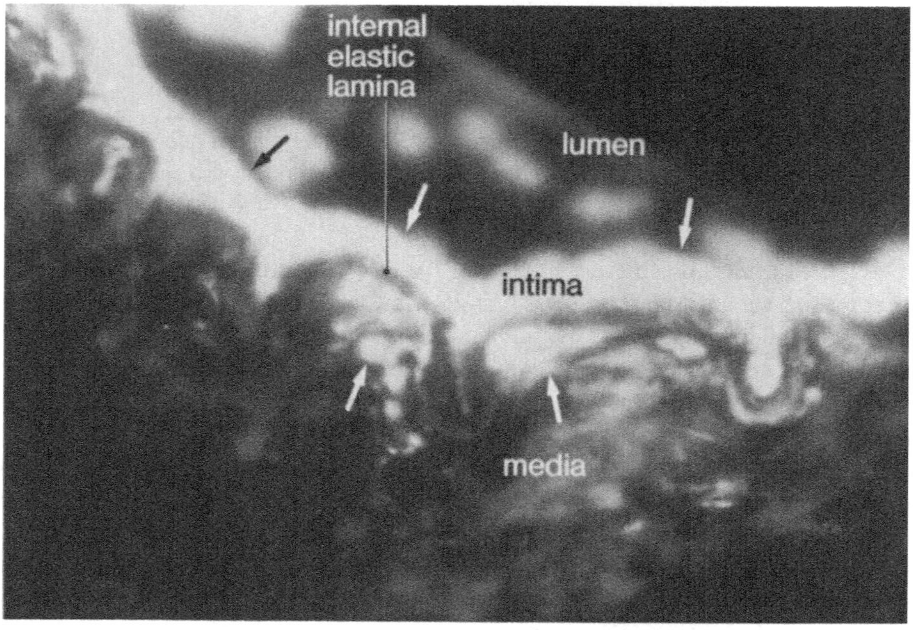

Fig. 114. Investigation of the IgG by an immunofluorescent study. IgG is observed in the intima and directly beneath the internal elastic lamina (*arrows*). (the proximal end of the middle cerebral artery). x 800

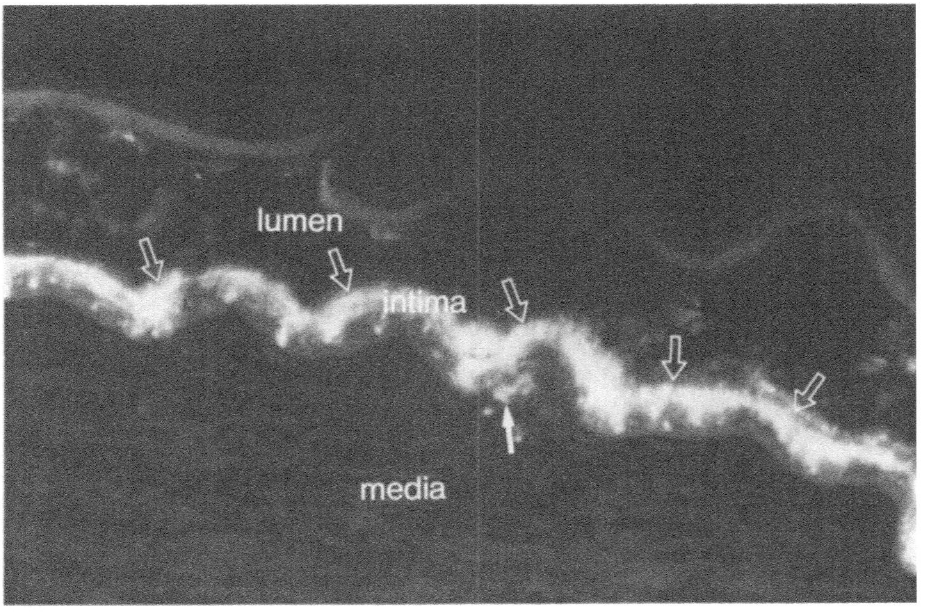

Fig. 115. Investigation of the IgM by an immunofluorescent study. Depositions of the IgM in the intima (⇨) and its slight spread into the media (➧) are observed (the terminal portion of the intracranial internal carotid artery). x 200

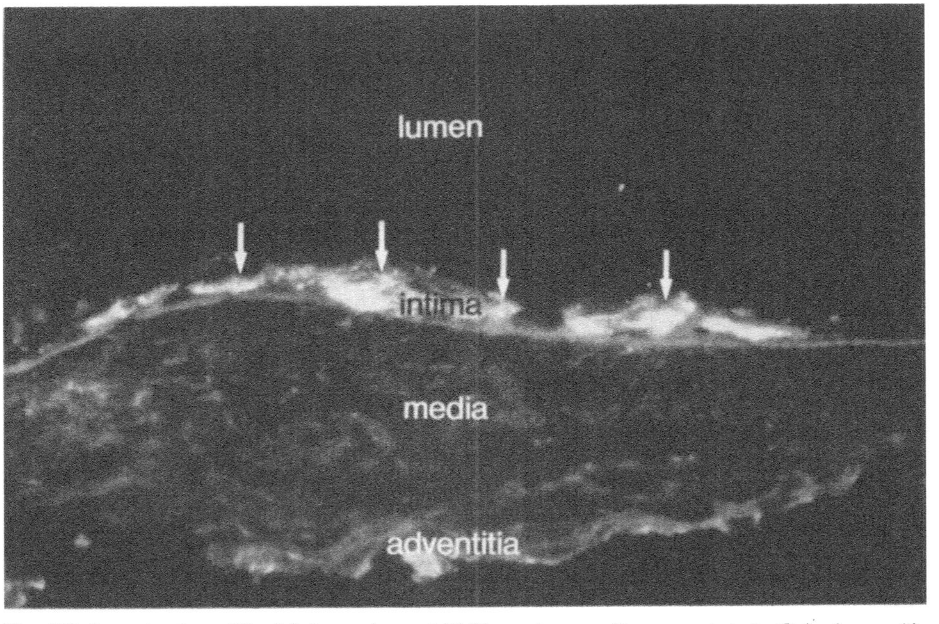

Fig. 116. Investigation of the third complement (C_3) by an immunofluorescent study. C_3 is observed in the intima (*arrows*). Fluorescence in the adventitia is due to nonspecific response (at the terminal portion of the intracranial internal carotid artery). x 200

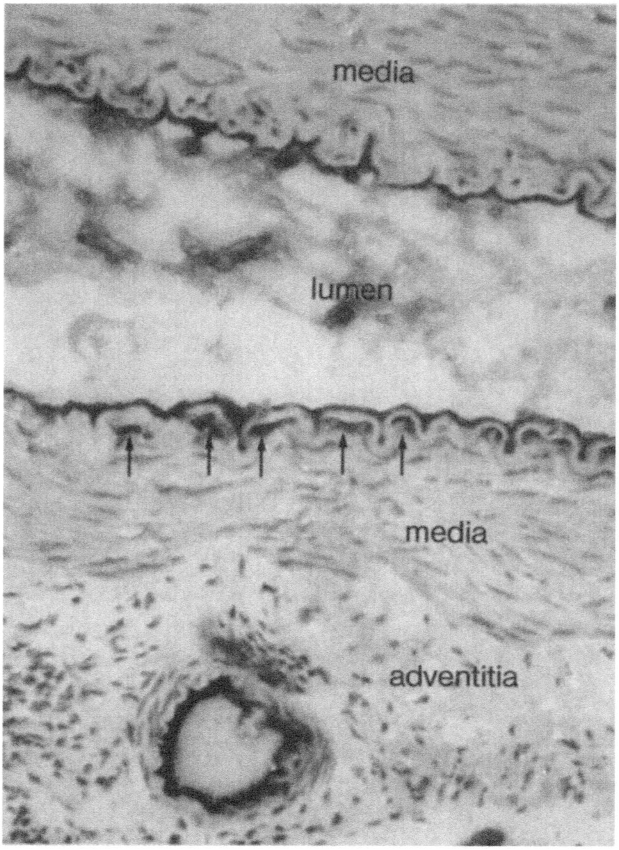

Fig. 117. Investigation of the antigen by an enzyme-antibody technique. The antibody is observed in the intima and directly beneath the internal elastic lamina (*arrows*) (the terminal portion of the intracranial internal carotid artery). x 200

some kind of local factor which puts certain vessels at greater risk to the immunological attack and subsequent pathological changes. Furthermore, it is known from various anatomical studies [260, 261] that the trunk arteries at the base of the brain around the terminal portion of the internal carotid artery receive dense sympathetic innervation from the superior cervical ganglion (SCG). If, therefore, the various organs in the neck region, such as the palatine tonsils and cervical lymph nodes, also receive sympathetic nerves from the SCG [194], then there could be retrograde stimulation of the sympathetic nerves due to heterologous protein produced at the site of inflammation in the neck region, i.e., by means of the so-called Reilly phenomenon [251, 347]. Since it is well known that the sympathetic nerves have a strong influence on the densely innervated regions of the trunk arteries of the brain and that vascular changes due to an

Table 22. Location and degree of cerebral arterial changes in general sensitization with right cervical lymph node stimulation. Severer cerebral arterial changes on the side of the sympathetic stimulation were seen in one out of three dogs whose lymph nodes near the superior cervical ganglion were stimulated by heterologous serum

No.		CIC	IC	M_1	A_1	PCOM	PC	$M_{2\text{-}5}$	$A_{2\text{-}5}$	BA
4	R	(+)	(+)	(+)	(−)	(−)	(−)	(−)	(−)	(−)
	L	(+)	(+)	(−)	(−)	(−)	(−)	(−)	(−)	(−)
5	R	(+++)	(−)	(−)	(−)	(+++)	(−)	(−)	(−)	(−)
	L	(+++)	(+)	(−)	(−)	(++)	(−)	(−)	(−)	(−)
6	R	(−)	(−)	(−)	(−)	(−)	(−)	(−)	(−)	(−)
	L	(−)	(−)	(−)	(−)	(−)	(−)	(−)	(−)	(−)

Abbreviations as for Table 20

immune reaction can be greatly aggravated by sympathetic nerve stimulation [234], the SCG was thought to be a strong candidate for the »local factor« responsible for the localization of the initial vascular changes in moyamoya disease.

Based upon these considerations, an experiment was undertaken, using the above canine model for systemic sensitization to antigen, in which direct stimulation of the cervical sympathetic nerves was done ipsilaterally.

Of the three dogs (Nos. 4–6) in which continuous stimulation of the sympathetic nerves near the SCG was done using heterologous protein, one showed mild vascular lesions and one showed severe changes only on the side of the sympathetic stimulation (Tables 19, 22). In five out of six dogs (Nos. 7–12) whose right SCGs were stimulated directly and continuously, localized vascular changes were observed and in three out of these five, more severe changes were

Table 23. Location and degree of cerebral arterial changes in general sensitization with right SCG stimulation. In five out of six dogs whose right SCGs were stimulated directly and continuously, localized vascular changes were observed. Moreover, in three out of these five dogs severer changes were seen on the side of the stimulation

No.		CIC	IC	M_1	A_1	PCOM	PC	$M_{2\text{-}5}$	$A_{2\text{-}5}$	BA
7	R	(−)	(+++)	(+)	(−)	(−)	(−)	(−)	(−)	(−)
	L	(−)	(−)	(−)	(−)	(−)	(−)	(−)	(−)	(−)
8	R	(−)	(++)	(−)	(−)	(−)	(−)	(−)	(−)	(−)
	L	(−)	(−)	(−)	(−)	(−)	(−)	(−)	(−)	(−)
9	R	(−)	(+++)	(−)	(−)	(−)	(−)	(−)	(−)	(−)
	L	(−)	(+)	(−)	(−)	(−)	(−)	(−)	(−)	(−)
10	R	(++)	(−)	(−)	(−)	(−)	(−)	(−)	(−)	(−)
	L	(++)	(−)	(−)	(−)	(−)	(−)	(−)	(−)	(−)
11	R	(−)	(+)	(−)	(−)	(−)	(−)	(−)	(−)	(−)
	L	(−)	(+)	(−)	(−)	(−)	(−)	(−)	(−)	(−)
12	R	(−)	(−)	(−)	(−)	(−)	(−)	(−)	(−)	(−)
	L	(−)	(−)	(−)	(−)	(−)	(−)	(−)	(−)	(−)

Abbreviations as for Table 20

Table 24. Location and degree of cerebral arterial changes in general sensitization with bilateral SCG stimulation. In three dogs whose bilateral SCGs were stimulated simultaneously, all three showed localized vascular changes bilaterally. In two out of these three dogs, the location and degree of vascular changes were similar on both sides

No.		CIC	IC	M_1	A_1	PCOM	PC	$m_{2\text{-}5}$	$A_{2\text{-}5}$	BA
13	R	(卌)	(卌)	(−)	(−)	(−)	(−)	(−)	(−)	(−)
	L	(+)	(+)	(−)	(−)	(−)	(−)	(−)	(−)	(−)
14	R	(+)	(+)	(−)	(−)	(−)	(−)	(−)	(−)	(−)
	L	(+)	(+)	(−)	(−)	(−)	(−)	(−)	(−)	(−)
15	R	(−)	(+)	(−)	(−)	(−)	(−)	(−)	(−)	(−)
	L	(−)	(+)	(−)	(−)	(−)	(−)	(−)	(−)	(−)

Abbreviations as for Table 20

found in the stimulated side (Tables 19, 23). To reconfirm these results, bilateral simultaneous stimulation of the SCG was carried out in three dogs (Nos. 13–15), and all three showed localized vascular pathology bilaterally, the sites and severity of which were similar on both sides in two animals (Table 19, 24). Finally, superior cervical ganglionectomy (SCG-ectomy) was performed unilaterally on the right side in six more dogs and continuous stimulation given to the remaining contralateral SCG (dogs. Nos. 16–21) (Tables 19, 25). In all six animals vascular changes confined to the vicinity of the terminal portion of the internal carotid artery were seen. Four of the dogs showed such lesions only on the side of the SCG stimulation, with no vascular changes on the side of the SCGectomy (Fig. 118). Of the two remaining dogs, one showed severe lesions only on the side of the sympathetic stimulation. In summary, SCGectomy resulted in the relative

Table 25. Location and degree of arterial changes in general sensitiziation with left SCG stimulation after right superior cervical ganglionectomy. In six dogs with right SCG ectomy all animals showed localized vascular changes. Four showed such lesions only on the side of the SCG stimulation, with no vascular changes on the side of the ganglionectomy

No.		CIC	IC	M_1	A_1	PCOM	PC	$M_{2\text{-}5}$	$A_{2\text{-}5}$	BA
16	R	(−)	(−)	(−)	(−)	(−)	(−)	(−)	(−)	(−)
	L	(#)	(卌)	(−)	(−)	(−)	(−)	(−)	(−)	(−)
17	R	(−)	(−)	(−)	(−)	(−)	(−)	(−)	(−)	(−)
	L	(−)	(#)	(−)	(−)	(−)	(−)	(−)	(−)	(−)
18	R	(−)	(#)	(−)	(−)	(−)	(−)	(−)	(−)	(−)
	L	(−)	(#)	(−)	(+)	(+)	(−)	(−)	(−)	(−)
19	R	(−)	(−)	(−)	(−)	(−)	(−)	(−)	(−)	(−)
	L	(−)	(+)	(−)	(−)	(−)	(−)	(−)	(−)	(−)
20	R	(−)	(−)	(−)	(−)	(−)	(−)	(−)	(−)	(−)
	L	(+)	(−)	(−)	(−)	(−)	(−)	(−)	(−)	(−)
21	R	(−)	(+)	(−)	(−)	(−)	(−)	(−)	(−)	(−)
	L	(−)	(+)	(−)	(−)	(−)	(−)	(−)	(−)	(−)

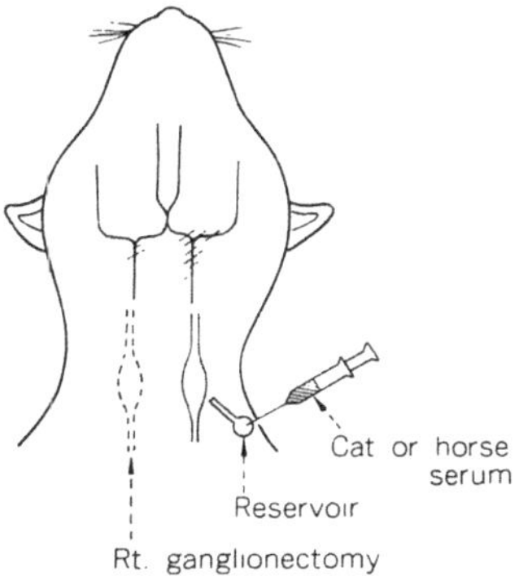

Fig. 118. Degree and location of the arterial change of the dog. After right superior cervical ganglionectomy, left SCG stimulation combined with general sensitization was performed. *Oblique line* shows the arterial change. More severe arterial changes were observed in the left side than in the right side

prevention of the vascular changes caused by the immune reaction in the denervated vessels of the majority of cases, as compared with the nontreated side, and when vascular changes were seen on the side of the SCGectomy they were milder than the changes ipsilateral to the intact SCG. These results strongly suggest the involvement of sympathetic nerves in the appearance and development of vascular changes due to an immune reaction mechanism.

11.4 Conclusion

Based upon the experimental results discussed in this chapter, we now believe that the causal mechanisms in moyamoya disease may be as follows.

First, due to a heterologous agent of some kind, there occurs inflammation of the organs of the neck (tonsils, cervical lymph nodes, etc.). This agent acts as an antigen and induces the production of antibody and immune complexes which then circulate throughout the body in the vascular system. Simultaneously, the antigen itself or the heterologous proteins produced at the site of inflammation stimulate the nearby sympathetic nerves. The SCG is then stimulated retrogradely. The permeability of the vessels receiving dense innervation from the SCG is caused to increase (from the intimal side), and the immune complexes in the bloodstream then enter the vascular walls, bringing about pathological changes. Subsequent development of thrombi in the vascular walls leads to hypertrophy of the intima, stenosis, and eventually vascular occlusion.

In this chapter the various hypotheses concerning moyamoya disease and our own experiments and hypothesis have been discussed. Definite progress has been made in clarifying the etiology of this disease, but it remains unclear why moyamoya disease is relatively so prevalent in Japanese and whether or not the juvenile and adult forms of the disease are due to the same factors and mechanisms.

12 Quasi-Moyamoya Diseases

12.1 Introduction

As discussed in earlier chapters, the angiographical diagnostic criteria for moyamoya disease are stenosis or occlusion of (a) the terminal portion of the bilateral internal carotid arteries (ICA), (b) the proximal portion of the anterior cerebral arteries (ACA), and (c) the middle cerebral arteries (MCA) due to unknown causes, together with an abnormal vascular network seen in the arterial phase in that region. Consequently, if these criteria are to be followed strictly, cases with stenosis of known cause or cases with unilateral abnormalities should not be considered to be true moyamoya disease.

In this chapter, we discuss those cases experienced by us which do not meet these strict criteria of true moyamoya disease, but which were cerebrovascular disorders similar to moyamoya disease. We will refer to these cases a »quasi-moyamoya disease,« in order to distinguish them from true moyamoya disease. Careful study of such cases is thought to be useful in the further clarification of the essential nature of true moyamoya disease.

12.2 Unilateral Quasi-Moyamoya Disease

12.2.1 Unilateral Quasi-Moyamoya Disease with Normal Contralateral Vessels

A variety of quasi-moyamoya disease cases have been reported in which the contralateral ICA was normal [161, 188, 203, 341]. Here we report upon two cases experienced by us.

Case 1: 44-year-old Male. The patient had contracted pleuritis at the age of 16 years and had suffered from hypertension from the age of 38 years.

At the age of 44 years, he experienced right hemiparesis without disturbance of consciousness. Some improvement in the hemiparesis was seen after 2 months, but at the time tremor of the right extremities began and, 8 months from onset of the right hemiparesis, he was admitted to our clinic for treatment (8 June 1973).

The neurological findings on admission were right hemiparesis and right intention tremor. Left carotid angiograms (CAGs) showed stenosis of the left ICA at the C_1 portion, stenosis of the left MCA at the M_1 portion, and stenosis of the left ACA at the A_1 portion. An abnormal vascular network was found around the left lenticulostriate arteries (Fig. 119). In right CAGs, no notable abnormalities were found (Fig. 120).

The case presented below was also a case of unilateral quasi-moyamoya disease, but with an associated cerebral aneurysm [325].

Case 2: 41-year-old Female. The patient was admitted to hospital after two attacks of subarachnoid hemorrhage in late September 1978.

There were no notable neurological findings on admission. Left CAGs showed occlusion of the C_1 portion of the ICA. The left MCA and the left ACA were not visualized, but the left PCA was visualized feeding from the left posterior communicating artery (PComA). Numerous collateral pathways were seen emerging from the left PCA. Although mild, a network of abnormal vessels was seen at the base of the brain near the region of stenosis (Fig. 121).

In right CAGs, there were no abnormalities near the terminal portion of the ICA, but an aneurysm of the anterior communicating artery (AComA) was apparent (Fig. 122). At the time of surgery, it was confirmed that the cause of the subarachnoid hemorrhage was in fact rupture of the cerebral aneurysm.

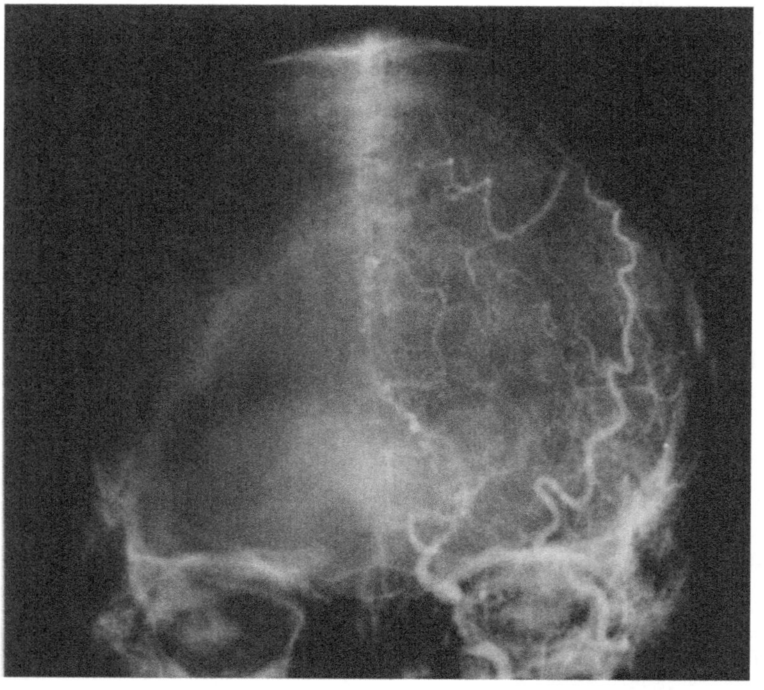

Fig. 119. Case 1: 41-year-old male. A case of unilateral quasi-moyamoya disease. Left carotid angiogram showed stenosis of the left C_1, M_1, and A_1, and moyamoya vessels at the base of the brain

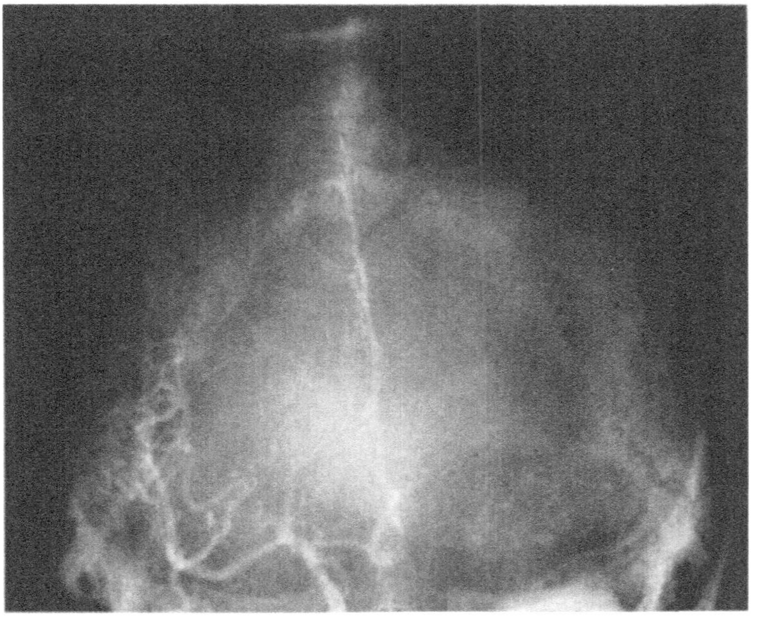

Fig. 120. Case 1: Right carotid angiogram without notable abnormalities

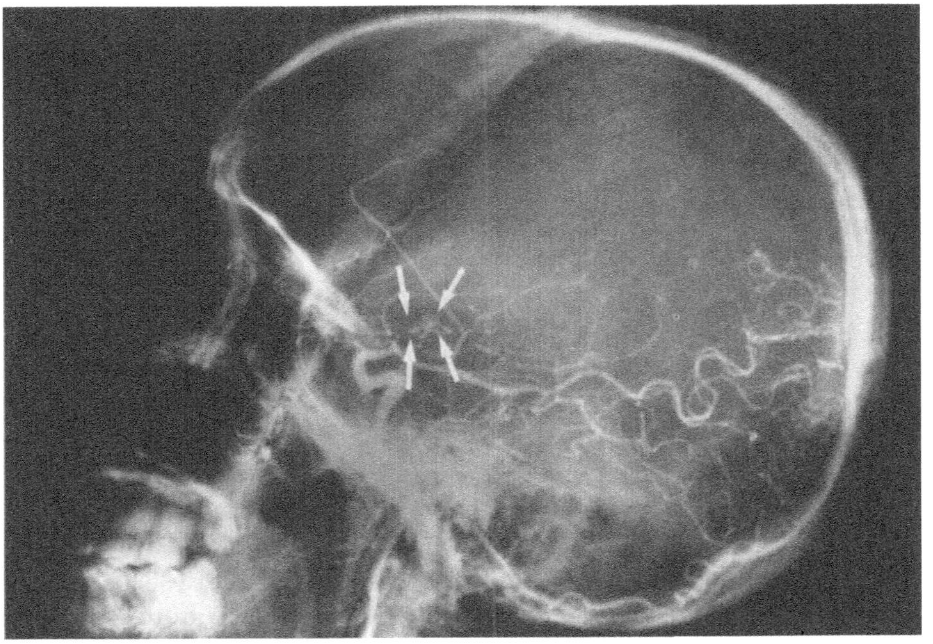

Fig. 121. Case 2: 41-year-old female. A case of unilateral quasi-moyamoya disease with aneurysm. Left carotid angiogram did not visualize the distal part from C_1 portion of the internal carotid artery, and mild moyamoya vessels (*arrows*) were recognized around it

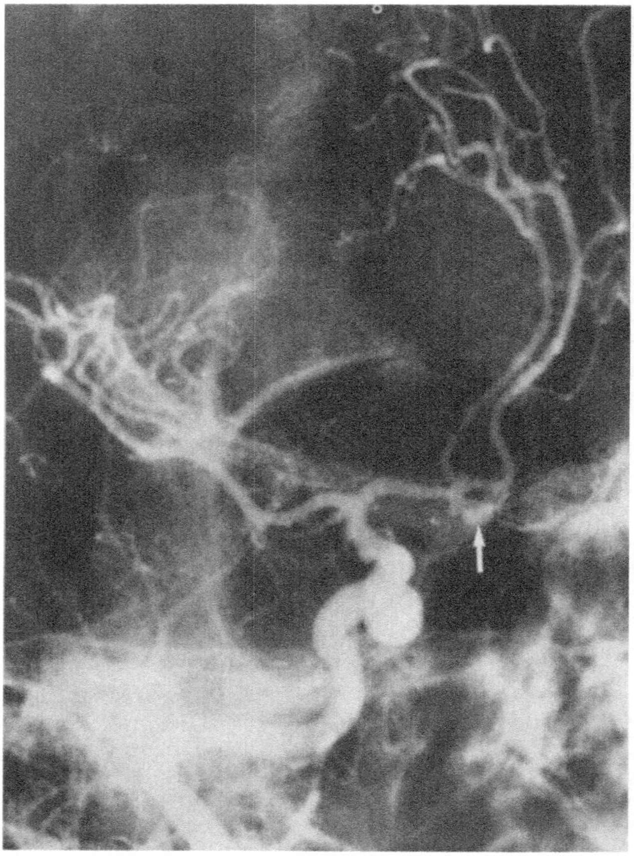

Fig. 122. Case 2 (the same case as in Fig. 121): Right carotid angiogram, oblique view, showed no abnormalities near the terminal portion of the internal carotid artery, but an aneurysm of the anterior communicating artery was apparent (*arrow*)

In this case, it was considered that the development and rupture of the aneurysm of the AComA was related to the increased blood flow to the left hemisphere from the right during ischemia.

12.2.2 Unilateral Quasi-Moyamoya Disease with Stenosis or Occlusion of the Contralateral MCA or ACA

There are some cases in which unilateral moyamoya-like vessels are found together with a normal contralateral ICA, but with stenosis or occlusion of the proximal portion of the contralateral MCA or ACA [32, 47, 144]. Here, a case of unilateral quasi-moyamoya disease with associated contralateral stenosis of the proximal portion of the ACA is presented.

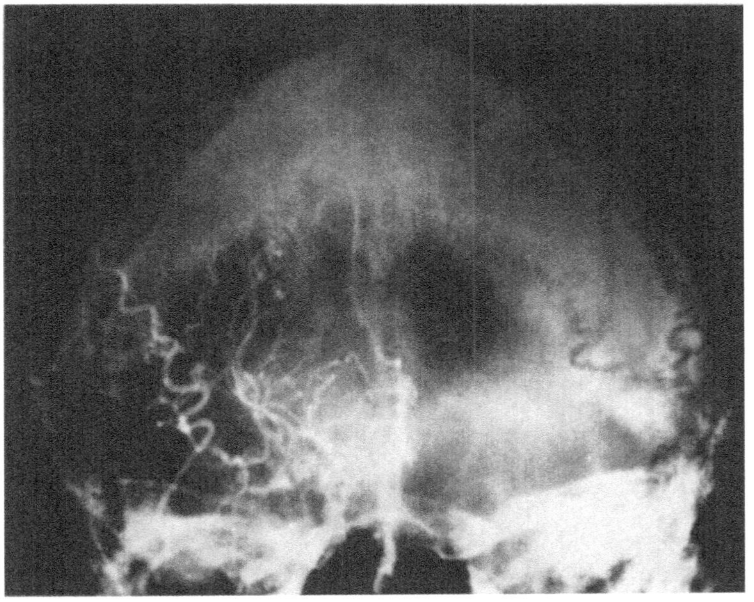

Fig. 123. Case 3: 24-year-old male. A case of quasi-moyamoya disease with stenosis of the contralateral anterior cerebral artery. Right carotid angiogram showed occlusion of the internal carotid artery at the C_1 portion and moyamoya vessels were seen arround the region

Case 3: 25-year-old Male. The patient suffered head trauma at the ages of 3 and 12 years and had a history of chronic tonsillitis. Between the ages of 13 and 15 years the patient experienced transient left hemiparesis on excessive exercise. At the age of 19 years, he sometimes experienced headache on excessive exercise and in July 1981 he was admitted to our clinic for further examination.

There were not notable neurological findings on admission. Right CAGs showed stenosis of the C_1 portion of the right ICA; the proximal portion of the ACA and the MCA were not visualized. An abnormal vascular network was seen around the region of stenosis. Through these abnormal vessels, a portion of the peripheral branches of the right ACA and MCA were seen (Fig. 123). In left CAGs, there were no abnormalities of the left ICA and left MCA, but there was stenosis of the proximal portion of the left ACA (Fig. 124). No abnormalities of the vertebrobasilar artery were seen, but collateral pathways developing from the right PComA were found (Fig. 125).

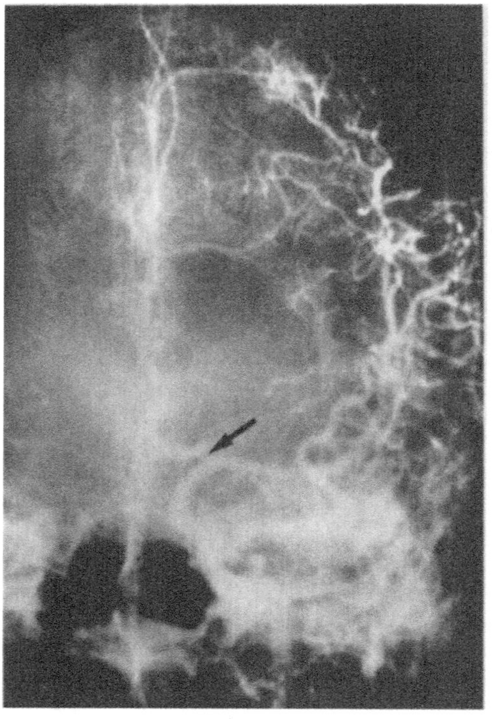

Fig. 124. Case 3 (the same case as in Fig. 123): Left carotid angiogram showed stenosis of the proximal portion of the left anterior cerebral artery (*arrow*)

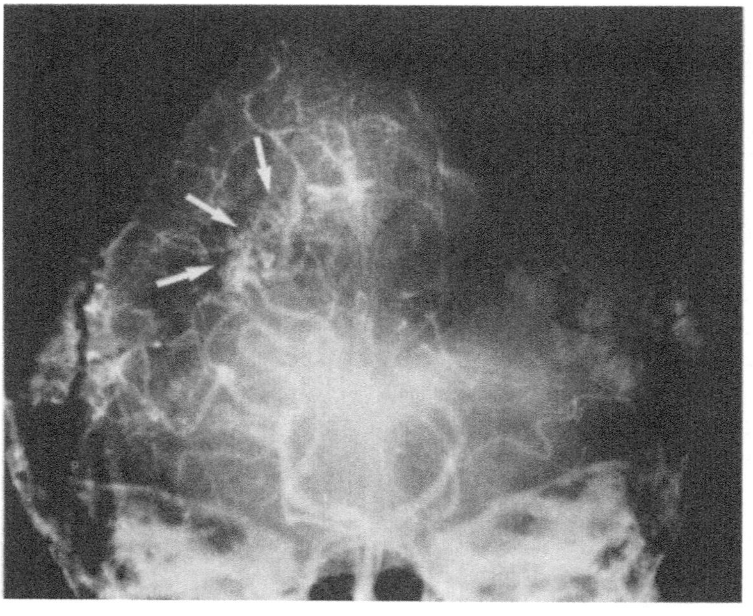

Fig. 125. Case 3 (the same case as in Figs. 123 and 124): Left vertebral angiogram showed collateral pathways developing to right frontal and temporal lobes (*arrows*)

12.3 Quasi-Moyamoya Disease in Which Bilateral or Unilateral Stenosis or Occlusion of the Proximal Portion of the MCA Is Seen, Together with Moyamoya Vessels in the Immediate Vicinity

It is thought that cases in which there is stenosis or occlusion of the proximal portion of the MCA and an abnormal vascular network nearby are not cases of true moyamoya disease based on the fact that there is no stenosis or occlusion of the terminal portion of the ICA or the ACA [44, 309, 325, 361].

Here a case in which there was unilateral stenosis of the proximal portion of the MCA together with moyamoya vessels surrounding it is presented.

Case 4: 40-year-old Male. The patient had experienced tonsillitis and from the age of 37 years had had hypertension. At the age of 36 years, he lost consciousness while drunk. Symptoms of the onset of the present illness were severe headache and nausea, and a lumbar puncture showed bloody liquor. On 31 October, 1975, he was admitted to hospital for emergency treatment.

On admission, he was delirious with a stiff neck. Bloody CSF and choked disks were seen, suggesting intracranial hypertension. Right CAGs showed occlusion of the proximal portion of the right MCA and an abnormal vascular network in the same region. The terminal portion of the MCA was visualized through these abnormal vessels (Fig. 126). Left carotid angiograms (CAGs) and left axillary vertebral (transaxillary) angiograms (A-VAGs) were normal. After instituting bilateral continuous ventricular drainage, a right intraventricular hematoma was discovered using Conray ventriculography (Fig. 127).

Unlike true moyamoya disease, the disease in this case is thought to have been the development of moyamoya vessels due to either a congenital vascular anomaly or the progression of arteriosclerotic stenosis in the proximal portion of the MCA. The cause of the intraventricular hemorrhage is thought to have been identical to that seen in other moyamoya disease cases.

12.4 Quasi-Moyamoya Disease with Vascular Malformations

Since congenital vascular anomalies cannot be ruled out in cases of moyamoya vessels with other associated cerebrovascular malformations, such cases are classified as quasi-moyamoya disease.

Here a case of quasi-moyamoya disease with a persistent primitive trigeminal artery is presented [237].

Case 5: 51-year-old Male. The patient had had tonsillitis as a child. At the age of 50 years, he occasionally suffered from lethargy and a dull headache.

One year later, on 18 October, 1979, he experienced a sudden headache and was hospitalized on the same day with some disturbance of consciousness and

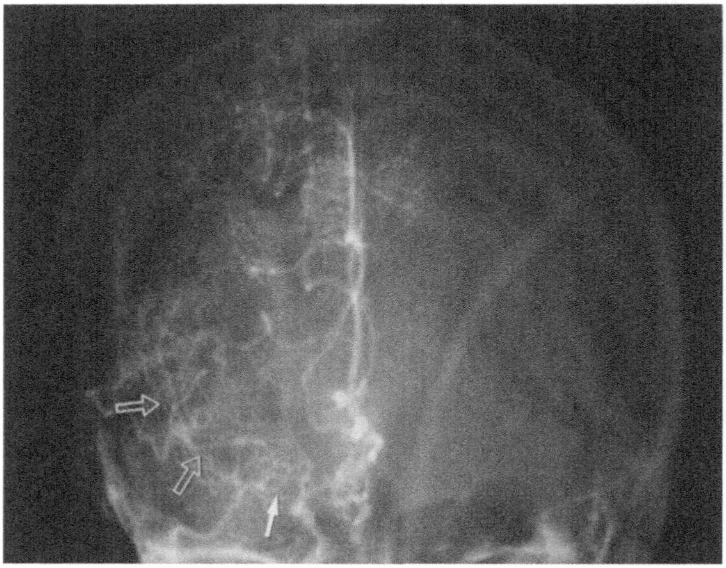

Fig. 126. Case 4: 40-year-old male. A case of quasi-moyamoya disease with unilateral occlusion of the middle cerebral artery. Right carotid angiogram showed occlusion of the proximal portion of the right middle cerebral artery (➧), and the terminal portion of the middle cerebral artery (⇨) was visualized through the moyamoya vessels

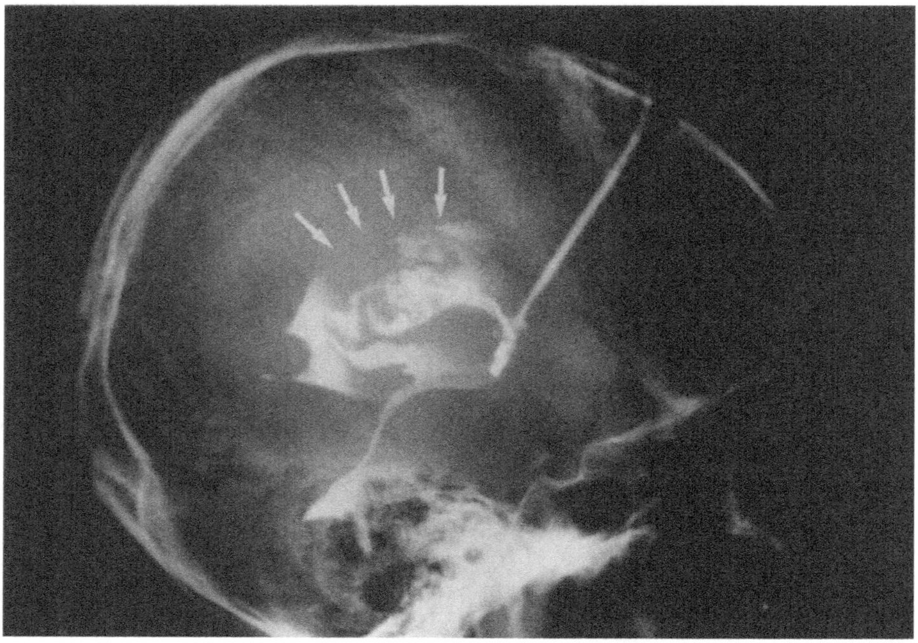

Fig. 127. Case 4 (the same case as in Fig. 126): Conray ventriculography showed the filling defect (*arrows*) due to right intraventricular hematoma

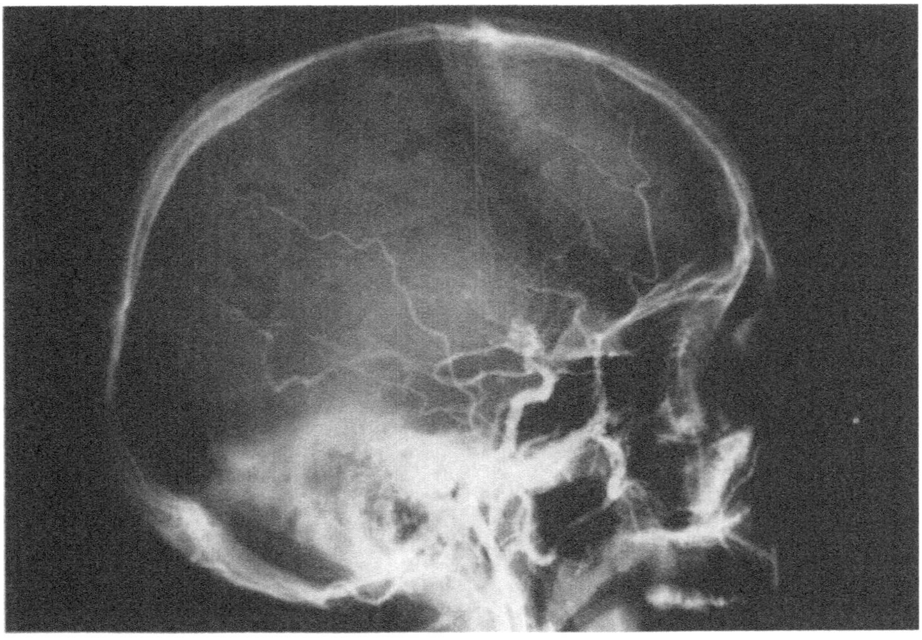

Fig. 128. Case 5: 51-year-old male. A case of quasi-moyamoya disease with persistent primitive trigeminal artery. Right carotid angiogram revealed irregularity of the lumen of the right internal carotid artery and occlusion at the C_1 portion. Moyamoya vessels were seen near the region of occlusion

right hemiparesis. Neurological findings on admission included a lethargic state of consciousness, aphasia (primarily sensory aphasia), and right hemiparesis. Right CAGs revealed irregularity of the lumen of the right ICA intracranially and occlusion at the C_1 portion. The proximal portion of the ACA and the MCA were not visualized and an abnormal vascular net was seen near the region of occlusion.

A portion of the peripheral MCA was found to be fed through this vascular net. Some collateral pathways from the right PComA and right PCA proceeding anteriorly were found (Fig. 128). In left CAGs, a persistent primitive trigeminal artery was seen. The bilateral superior cerebellar arteries and PCAs, as well as abundant collateral pathways, were visualized through the persistent primitive trigeminal artery. At the syphon of the left ICA, there was irregularity of the vascular lumen and there was abnormal elevation and stenosis of the C_1 portion. At the base of the brain, there was an abnormal vascular network. Peripheral branches of the left ACA and MCA were visualized through these collateral pathways (Fig. 129).

Computerized tomographic findings on the 6th day from onset included a high-density region and perifocal low-density extending from the left temporal lobe to the parietal lobe. These findings were presumed to be due to the intracerebral hematoma (Fig. 130).

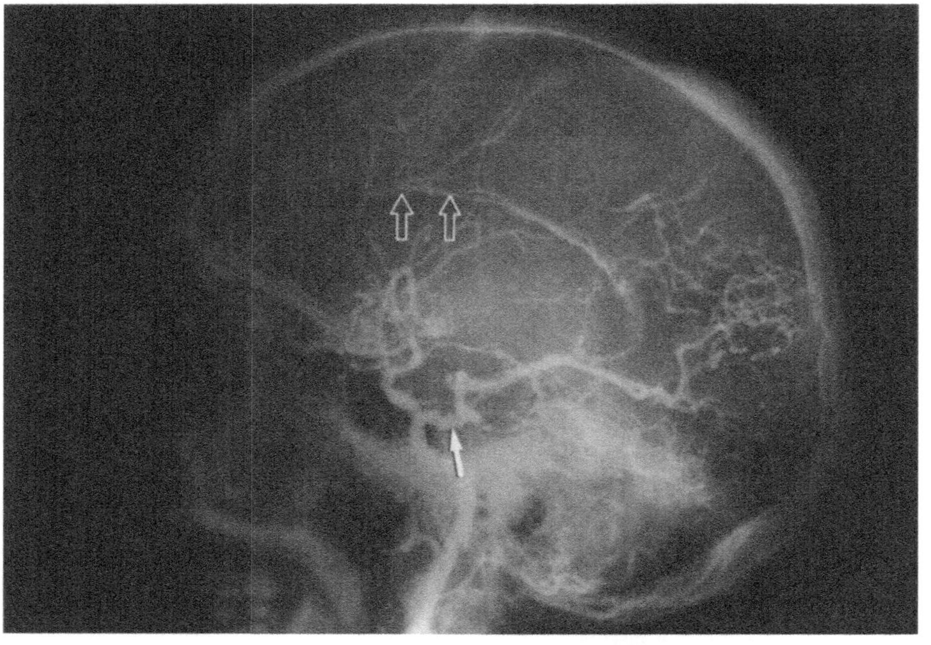

Fig. 129. Case 5 (the same case as Fig. 128): Left carotid angiogram showed irregularity of the lumen at the terminal portion of the left internal carotid artery and occlusion at the C_1 portion (➧). Also, the peripheral branches of the anterior cerebral artery were visualized through the posterior cerebral artery fed from the persistent primitive trigeminal artery which originated from the C_4–C_5 border portion (⇨)

For the following reasons, the vascular anomalies in this case were thought to be due either to arteriosclerotic vascular occlusion or to congenital occlusion of the ICA associated with the persistent primitive trigeminal artery. First, it was evident that moyamoya vessels at the base of the brain and bilateral occlusion of the terminal portion of the ICA were associated with a known congenital lesion, the persistent primitive trigeminal artery remaining from the fetal stage. Second, severe irregularities of the lumen of the ICA were notable bilaterally. Third, the ethmoidal and vault moyamoya vessels, which are usually well developed in true moyamoya disease, were absent.

12.5 Quasi-Moyamoya Disease Due to Known Causes

There are various cases presenting a moyamoya-like appearance in cerebral angiograms, but in which the presence of a causal lesion, such as brain tumor [92, 254], trauma, or inflammation, is clearly evident.

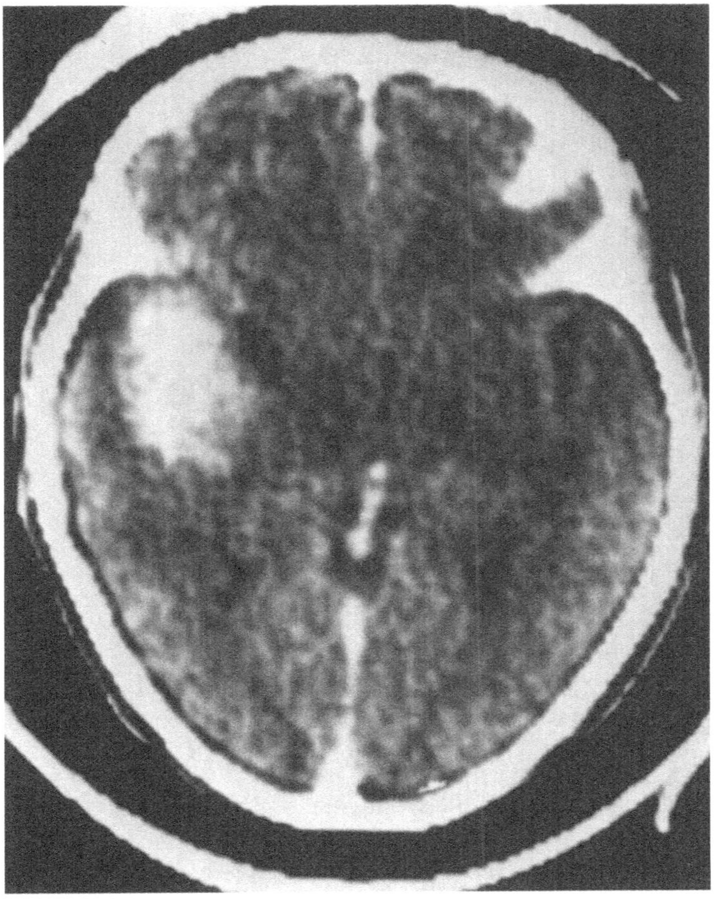

Fig. 130. Case 5 (the same case as in Figs. 128 and 129: CTscan showed the intracerebral hematoma in the left temporal lobe

12.5.1 Quasi-Moyamoya Disease Associated with von Recklinghausen's Disease

It is well known that some cases of von Recklinghausen's disease present an angiographical appearance similar to moyamoya disease [72, 157, 179, 330]. Over the past 10 years, we have experienced 32 cases of von Recklinghausen's disease, 3 of which had moyamoya-like vessels. All three cases had cerebral tumors, but in only one of these cases was there the suggestion of direct compression of the terminal portion of the ICA due to the tumor.

Below, two of these cases — one in which direct compression by the tumor was found and one in which such compression was not found — are presented.

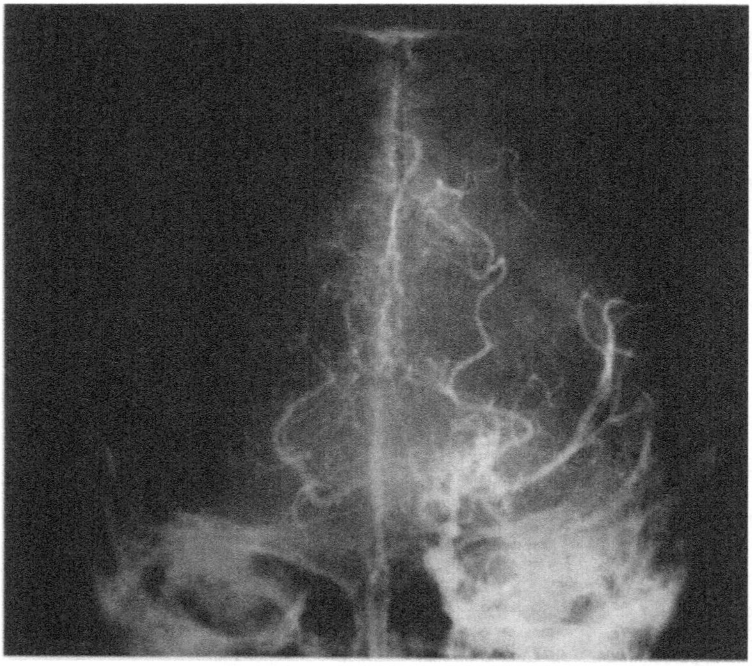

Fig. 131. Case 6: 37-year-old male. Quasi-moyamoya disease with von Recklinghausen's disease. Left carotid angiogram showed the stenosis at C_1, M_1, and A_1, and the development of moyamoya vessels in this region

Case 6: 37-year-old Male. The patient's eldest daughter had had luxation of the hip joint and café au lait spots. From infancy, the patient showed café au lait spots on the skin and, at the age of 33 years, subcutaneous tumors were diagnosed. From the age of 35 years, he complained of attacks of frontalgia, dizziness, and nausea.

On 10 February, 1975, at the age of 37 years, he was admitted to our clinic for detailed examination.

Neurological findings on admission included olfactory disturbance and right facial paresis. Café au lait spots were found on the skin over the entire body and the presence of subcutaneous neurofibroma was confirmed.

Angiographically, the frontal aspect of the right CAGs revealed stenosis of the terminal portion of the A_1 region of the ACA and a small abnormal vascular network in that vicinity. There was elevation of the peripheral A_1 portion and a leftward shift of the peripheral A_2 portion. In the lateral aspect, round displacement of the A_2 portion in a posterior direction was seen. In left CAGs, the C_1 portion of the left ICA was found to be stenotic and there was a lateroposterior shift in the M_2 portion. The left ACA was markedly stenotic and it fed an abnormal vascular network. The A_2 portion was incompletely visualized and there was posterior displacement of the left ACA, similar to that seen on the right (Figs. 131, 132). In the Left A-VAGs, the development of collateral pathways in

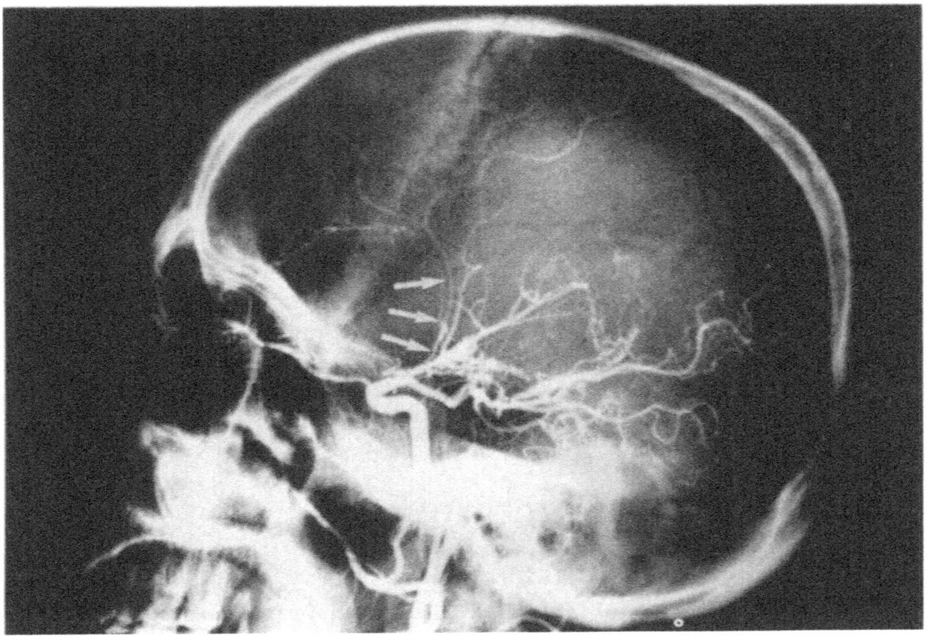

Fig. 132. Case 6 (the same case as in Fig. 131): Left carotid angiogram showed posterior displacement of the A_2 portion of the anterior cerebral artery (*arrows*)

an anterior direction was seen through the posterior pericallosal artery. In light of these angiographical findings and those of brain scintigrams (Fig. 133), a diagnosis was made of quasi-moyamoya disease developing due to the compression by the tumor at the center of the frontal fossa.

Case 7: 10-year-old Female. From the age of 6 years, the patient had shown café au lait spots on the face and subcutaneous neurofibromas were found on the body and face. From the age of 9 years, she experienced frontalgia, occasionally accompanied by nausea. At the age of 10 years, right hearing disturbance developed. She was admitted to hospital for further examination of 28 July, 1969.

Neurological findings on admission included disturbance of cranial nerves V, VII, and VIII on the left side. Angiographically, bilateral stenosis of the C_2 portion of the ICA and moyamoya vessels were found in both left and right CAGs (Fig. 134). The patient had a right cerebellopontine angle tumor and subtotal removal was performed. No direct relationship between the tumor and the above-mentioned vascular anomalies was evident.

In von Recklinghausen's disease, there are not only skin lesions, but also abnormalities of the bone and dura mater, and there are also reports of pathological findings of blood vessels [157, 257, 330]. It is thought that in the

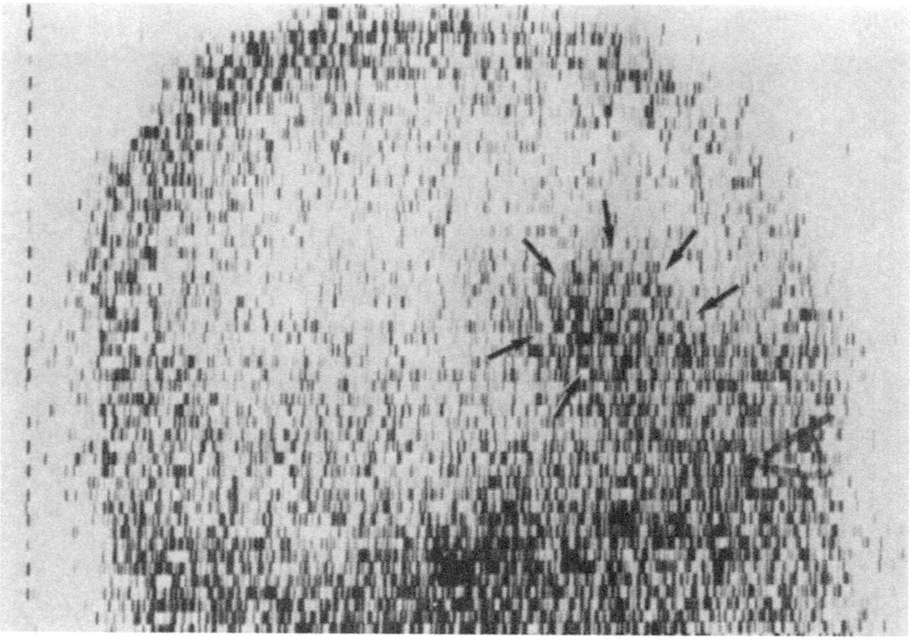

Fig. 133. Case 6 (the same case as in Figs. 131 and 132: Brain scintigram showed the tumor shadow at the base of the brain (*arrows*)

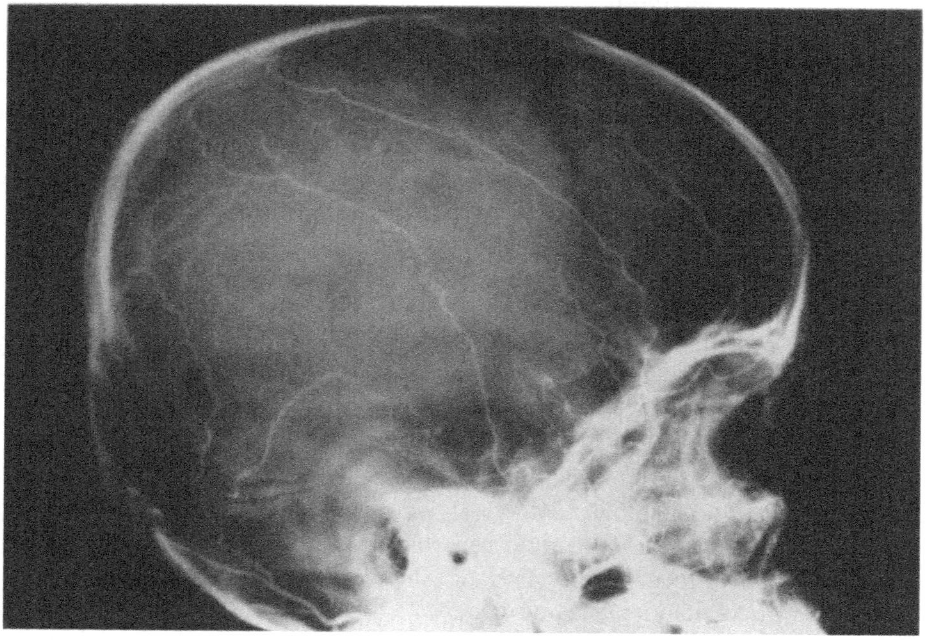

Fig. 134. Case 7: 10-year-old female. A case of quasi-moyamoya disease with von Recklinghausen's disease. Right carotid angiogram showed occlusion of the C_2 portion of the internal carotid artery, and moyamoya vessels near the lesion were seen bilaterally

present case the moyamoya vessels may have developed as a result of the stenosis and occlusion of the terminal portion of the bilateral ICA due, presumably, to such vascular anomalies.

12.5.2 Quasi-Moyamoya Disease Seen After Injury to Cerebral Arteries Caused by Trauma

It is known that stenosis or occlusion of the vessels near the terminal portion of the ICA [350] can occur due to mechanically induced cerebral vasospasm [13] following head trauma. Subsequently, moyamoya vessels have been found to develop in that region. From angiographical follow-up of such cases, it is known that the moyamoya vessels in some cases disappear, whereas in other cases the abnormal vascular network develops in a manner extremely similar to true moyamoya disease [233]. Examples of both types of lesions are presented below.

Case 8: 12-year-old Female. The patient had had tonsillitis. On 23 October, 1972, she suffered a blow to the right temporal region. She did not lose consciousness, but 2 h later she experienced headache and 24 h later she had left hemiparesis. She was then brought to our clinic.

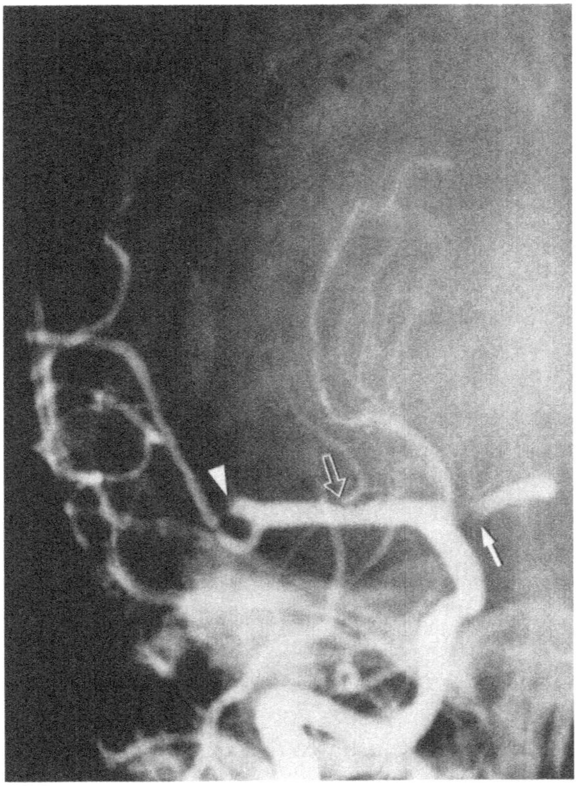

Fig. 135. Case 8: 12-year-old female. A case of quasi-moyamoya disease seen transiently after injury to cerebral arteries caused by trauma. Right carotid angiogram showed filling defect of the proximal portion of the right anterior cerebral artery (➽), irregularities of the walls of the right M_1 (⇩), and occlusion of M_2 (▶)

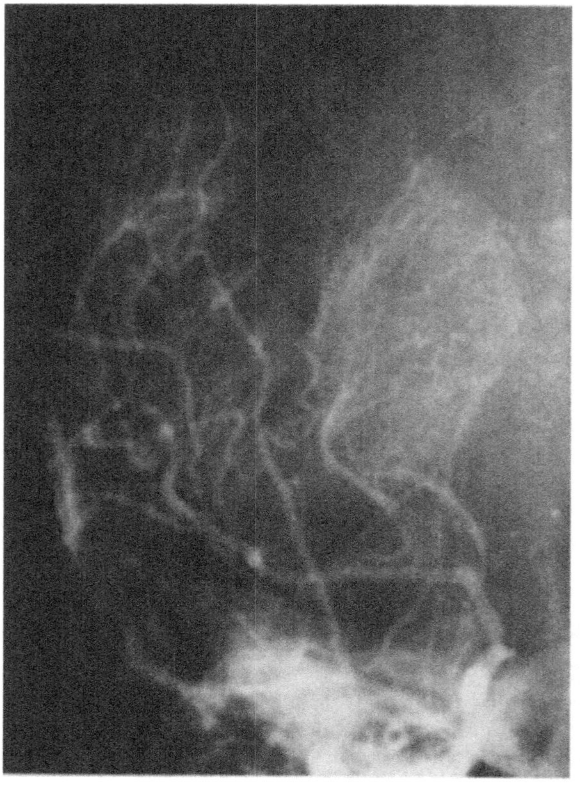

Fig. 136. Case 8 (the same case as in Fig. 135): Follow-up right carotid angiogram taken 18 days after the onset of disease showed stenosis at the distal portion from C_2 and moyamoya vessels at the regions of the basal ganglia

Neurological findings on admission included left hemiparesis, but consciousness was clear. Right CAGs on admission showed a shadow defect of the proximal portion of the right ACA extending over 3 mm and irregularities of the walls of the middle portion of the right M_1. Approximately 5 mm peripheral from the bifurcation of the right MCA, one of the M_2 branches was occluded (Fig. 135). In left CAGs, there were no notable abnormalities and the bilateral ACAs were visualized from the left.

Improvement of symtoms was found following procaine blocks of the cervical sympathetic ganglion, Urokinase therapy, right superior cervical ganglionectomy (SCGectomy), and perivascular sympathectomy (PVSectomy) at the bifurcation of the common carotid artery.

In the right CAGs taken 18 days from onset, stenosis of the entire MCA, the C_1 and C_2 portions of the ICA, and the proximal A_1 portion of the ACA was found, but the vascular occlusion previously seen was no longer present. There was abnormal dilatation of the lenticulostriate arteries and the development of moyamoya-like vessels (Fig. 136).

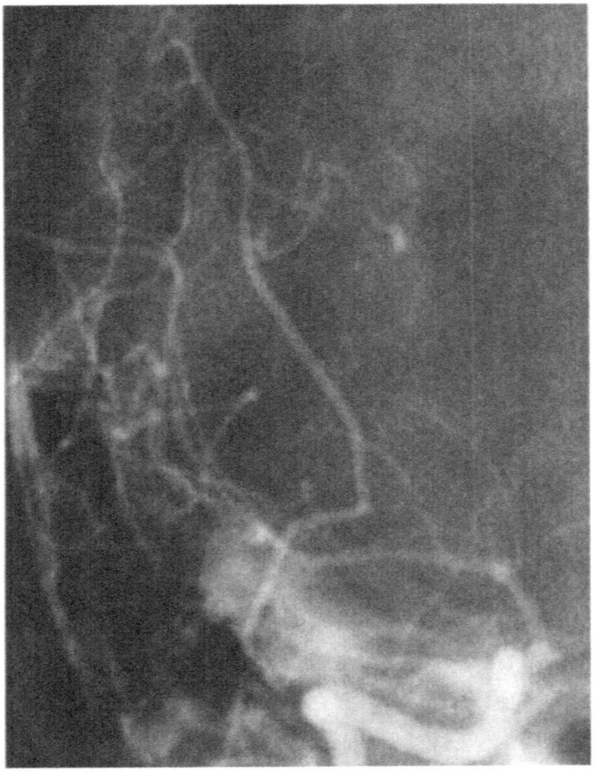

Fig. 137. Case 8 (the same case as in Figs. 135 and 136): Follow-up right carotid angiogram taken 1 month after onsset of disease showed that the vascular stenosis was unchanged, but moyamoya vessels were no longer evident

Right CAGs taken 1 month from onset showed that the vascular stenosis was unchanged, but the moyamoya-like vessels were no longer evident (Fig. 137). In right CAGs taken 5 months from onset, the stenosis had also disappeared and a nearly normal vascular appearance was found (Fig. 138).

Case 9: 28-year-old Male. The patient had had frequent fevers due to tonsillitis as a child. On 20 December, 1979, he was hit by a car while crossing the road in a drunken state. He was carried 8 m on the hood of the car before striking the left side of his head on the road. He lost consciousness immediately and was brought to our clinic some 40 min later.

Findings on admission included cuts over the left frontal and left temporal regions and swelling of the left clavicular region. His state of consciousness was judged as semicomatose. Right hemiparesis was found together with acceleration of deep reflexes and pathological reflexes on the right. There were no abnormalities of the light reflex or ocular fundus, but a large left-sided anisocoria was found.

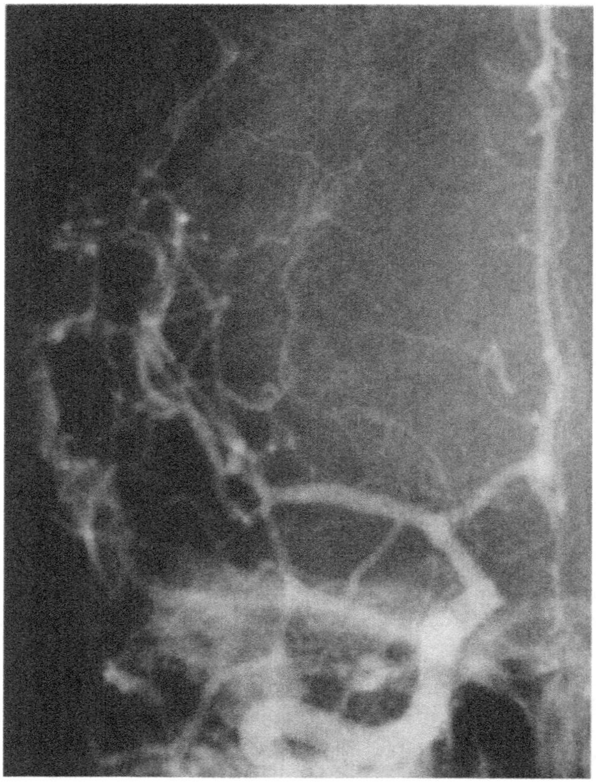

Fig. 138. Case 8 (the same cases as in Figs. 135–137):. Follow-up right carotid angiogram taken 5 months after the onset of disease showed disappearance of moyamoya vessels and a nearly normal vascular appearance

On X-ray films of the skull, linear fractures of the left temporal and left parietal bones were apparent. Left CAGs taken 2 h following the trauma gave no findings suggestive of intracranial hematoma, but there was marked stenosis of the vicinity of the terminal portion of the ICA, particularly at the proximal portion of the M_1 (Fig. 139). Right CAGs taken at the same time showed stenosis of the terminal portion of the ICA and the proximal portion of the M_1. The entire A_1 portion was narrow and none of the peripheral branches of the A_2 portion were visualized (Fig. 140).

At follow-up, left CAGs, progressive stenosis of the C_1, M_1, and A_1 portions were seen 6 days from the initial injury (Fig. 139), and those portions of the A_2 were barely visible. There was also a midline shift to the right. After 1 month (Fig. 139), the stenosis had further progressed and the A_1 and M_1 portions were visualized only as narrow, indistinct threads. None of the peripheral branches of the M_2 portion were seen. In a lateral view, the C_1, C_2, $M_1$and A_1 portions showed progressive narrowing and there was the development of moyamoya vessels in the immediate vicinity.

Follow-up CAGs gave only slight visualization of bilateral MCA branches at 42 days after the trauma (Fig. 140). There was also the appearance of moyamoya

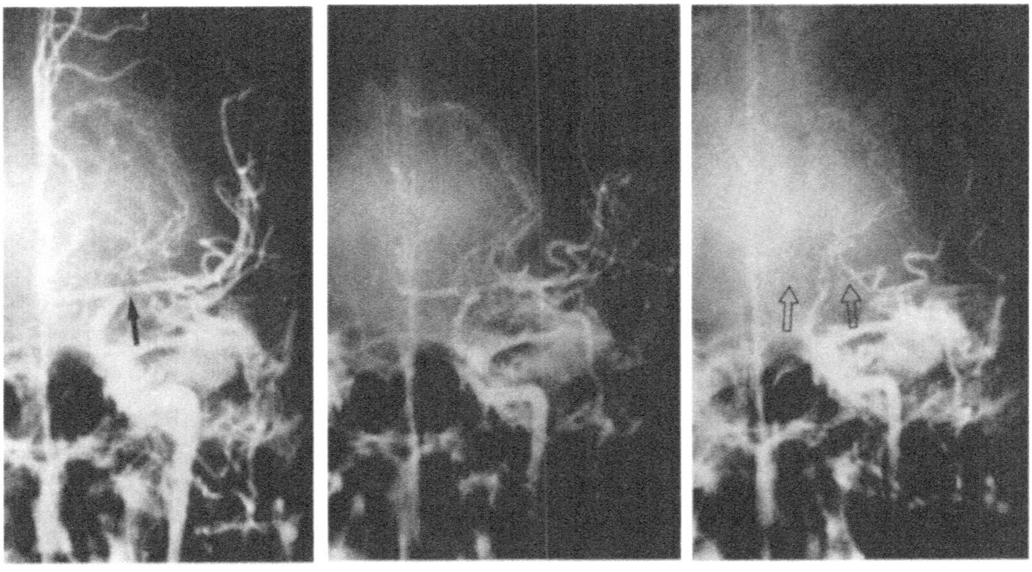

Fig. 139. Case 9: 28-year-old male. A case of advancing quasi-moyamoya disease seen after head trauma. Left carotid angiogram taken 2 h following the trauma (*left*) showed marked stenosis of the carotid fork, particularly at the proximal portion of the M_1 (➧). The follow-up angiogram 6 days later (*center*) showed progressive stenosis of the C_1, M_1, and A_1, and there was the development of moyamoya vessels. After 1 month (*right*), the stenosis had progressed further and the A_1 and M_1 portions were visualized only as narrow as thread (⇨), and peripheral branches of the M_2 portion were not seen

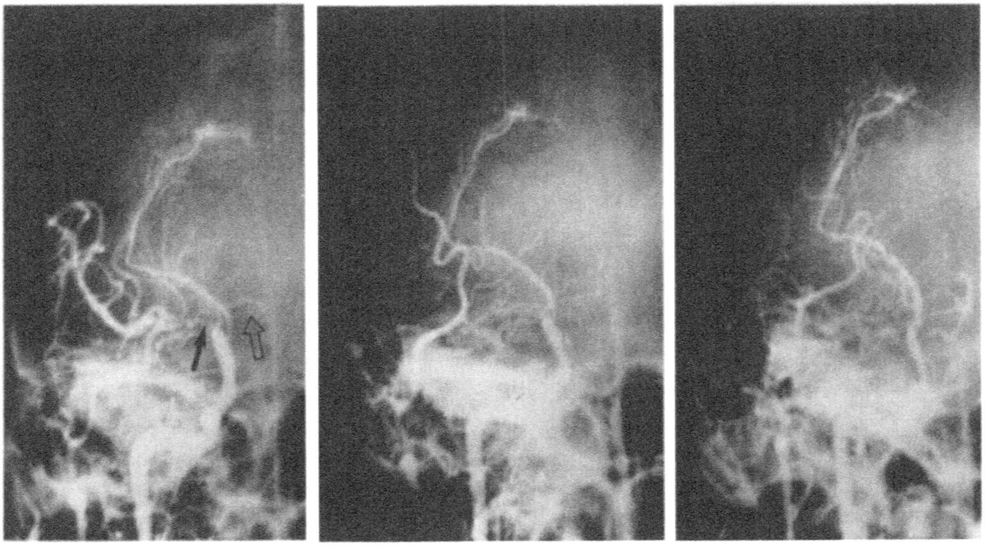

Fig. 140. Case 9 (the same case as in Fig. 139): Right carotid angiogram taken 2 h following the traume (*left*) showed stenosis of the proximal portion of the M_1 (➧) and the entire A_1 portion was narrow (⇨) and peripheral branches of the A_2 portion were not visualized. Follow-up angiogram of 42 days after the trauma (*center*) showed only slight visualization of branches of the middle cerebral artery and the emergence of moyamoya vessels. After 5 months (*right*) the development of moyamoya vessels was seen

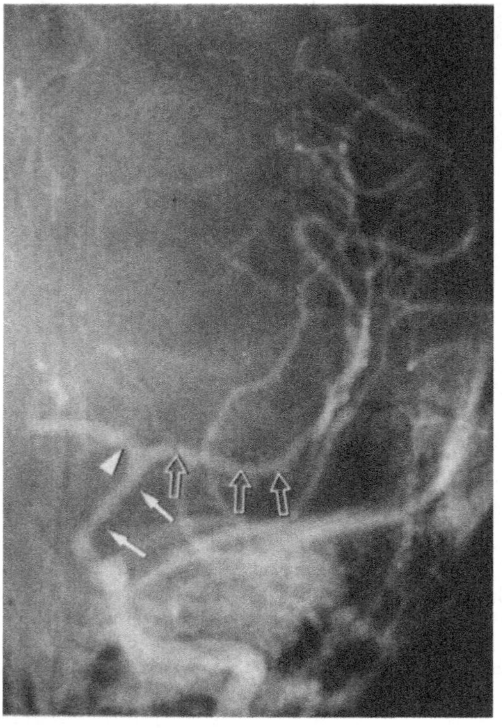

Fig. 141. Case 10: 8-year-old male. A case of quasi-moyamoya disease with fibromuscular dysplasia. Left carotid angiogram taken 7 days after onset revealed stenosis of the C_1, C_2 (➽), and A_1 (▶). There was also a »string of beads« appearance at the M_1 and M_2 (⇨) portions

vessels thought to be developments of the perforators at the base of the brain. After 5 months (Fig. 140), an enlarged anterior choroidal artery could be seen, together with the proliferation of moyamoya vessels.

12.5.3 Quasi-Moyamoya Disease Associated with Fibromuscular Dysplasia

Fibromuscular dysplasia is a rare stenotic lesion with a predilection for the renal arteries and the cervical portion of the ICA, but there have also been reports of its occurrence on intracranial vessels [247], especially the proximal portion of the MCA. Angiograms of fibromuscular dysplasia reveal a characteristic »string of beads« appearance [87] along the lumen of the affected vessels due to irregular stenosis and dilatation.

Next, a case of a boy with moyamoya-like angiographical findings who also showed gradual progression of vascular stenosis which was thought to be due to fibromuscular dysplasia is presented.

Case 10: 8-year-old Male. The patient had experienced several asthma-like attacks.

On 4 December, 1972, he suffered sudden clonic convulsions of the right side of his body while eating lunch. Thirty minutes later he lost consciousness. After

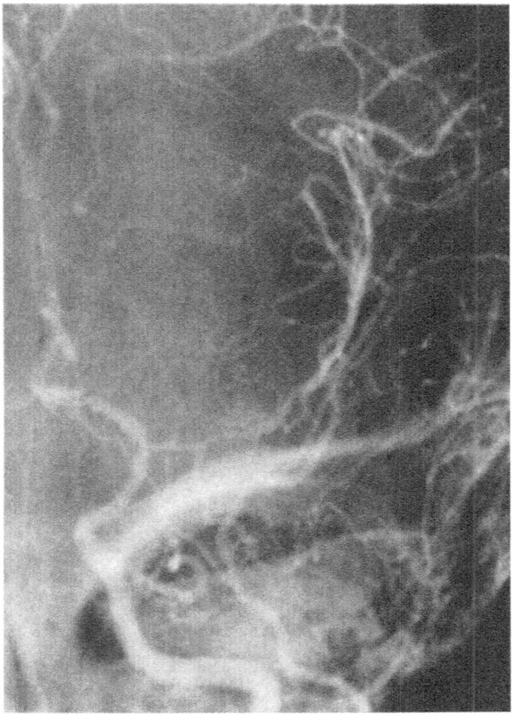

Fig. 142. Case 10 (the same case as in Fig. 141): Left carotid angiogram taken 3 months later showed progressive stenosis especially at the portion of the M_1

regaining consciousness, he had right hemiparesis and aphasia, and was brought to our clinic 2 days later.

Neurological findings on admission included right hemiparesis and motor aphasia, although consciousness was normal. Left CAGs taken 7 days from onset showed mild stenosis of the C_1 portion of the left ICA and of the proximal A_1 portion of the left ACA. There was also irregularity of the lumen of the M_1 and M_2 portions of the left MCA, which showed the characteristic »string of beads« appearance (Fig. 141).

Left CAGs taken 3 months later showed narrowing of the bifurcation of the left ICA and the entire M_1 portion, with the »string of beads« sign still apparent at the proximal portion of the M_2 (Fig. 142).

Eight months later, left CAGs revealed moderate stenosis of the A_1 portion and the C_1, C_2 portions of the ICA. Marked stenosis was seen on the left MCA from the M_1 to the M_2 portions (Fig. 143). After 20 months, left CAGs revealed severe stenosis at the bifurcation of the ICA and the proximal region of the ACA. The proximal portion of the MCA was occluded and the peripheral M_1 and M_2 regions were well visualized through a small network of moyamoya vessels in that region (Fig. 144).

In right CAGs, the ICA was seen to be normal, and there was sufficient visualization of the left ACA through the AComA.

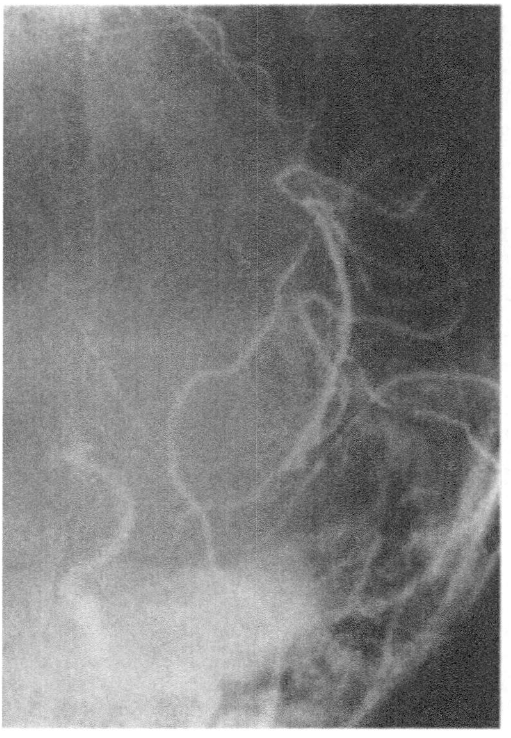

Fig. 143. Case 10 (the same case as in Fig. 142): Left carotid angiogram taken 8 months later showed that stenosis of the M_1 and A_1 portions was more advanced and their peripheral branches were less visualized

12.5.4 Quasi-Moyamoya Disease Due to Tuberculous Vasculitis

There are some cases showing moyamoya-like vessels in angiograms secondary to tuberculous meningitis or vasculitis [171]. Here a case with a history of tuberculous meningitis is reported.

Case 11: 10-year-old Female. At the age of 5 years, the patient contracted tuberculous meningitis. On 29 September, 1961, she was hit in the right frontal region with a soft mass of dirt. She had a loss of memory of approximately 20 s during these events. Forty minutes later, she experienced left hemiparesis and consciousness became drowsy. She was then hospitalized.

Right CAGs revealed a rostral displacement of the ACA, severe stenosis of the terminal syphon portion of the ICA, and moyamoya vessels in the immediate vicinity. The MCA was only barely visible (Fig. 145).

Craniotomy and removal of the hematoma were performed immediately, but the patient died 3 days postoperatively. Autopsy revealed an already healed tubercle and diffuse intimal thickening of cerebral vessels. There was marked neovascularization in the region of the MCA.

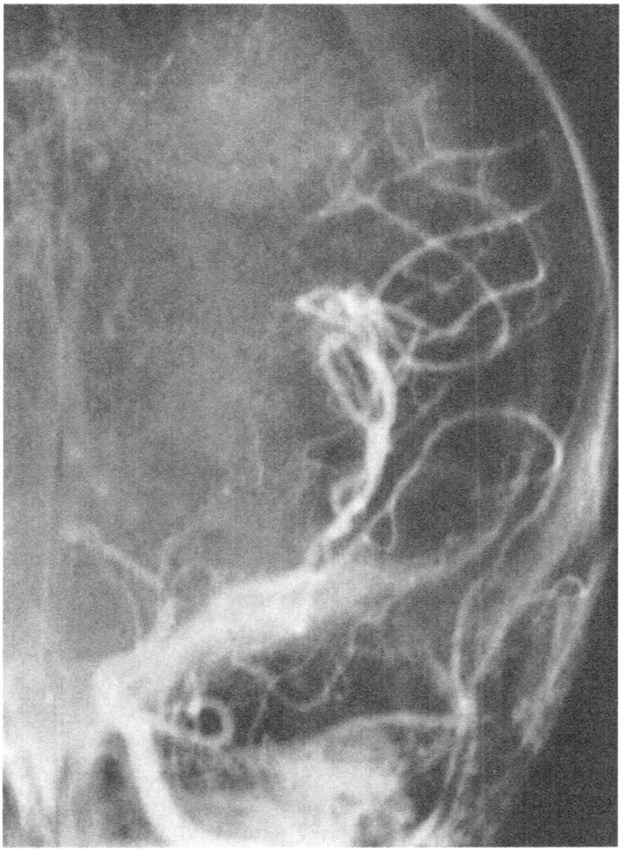

Fig. 144. Case 10 (the same case as in Figs. 141–143): Left carotid angiogram taken 20 months later revealed severe stenosis at the C_1 and A_1 portions. The proximal portion of the M_1 was occluded and moyamoya vessels were seen in this region

12.6 Quasi-Moyamoya Disease Due to Other Causes

There have been various reports concerning other varieties of quasi-moyamoya disease. These include: quasi-moyamoya disease due to cerebral arteriosclerosis [73, 249]; quasi-moyamoya disease developing subsequent to radiation therapy [250, 264]; quasi-moyamoya disease associated with Fanconi's anemia [26]; quasi-moyamoya disease with sickle cell anemia [154, 263, 277]; quasi-moyamoya disease due to obsolete, generalized, nonspecific arteritis [210]; quasi-moyamoya disease with associated connective tissue disorders [253]; and quasi-moyamoya disease due to cerebral angitis caused by leptospirosis [343].

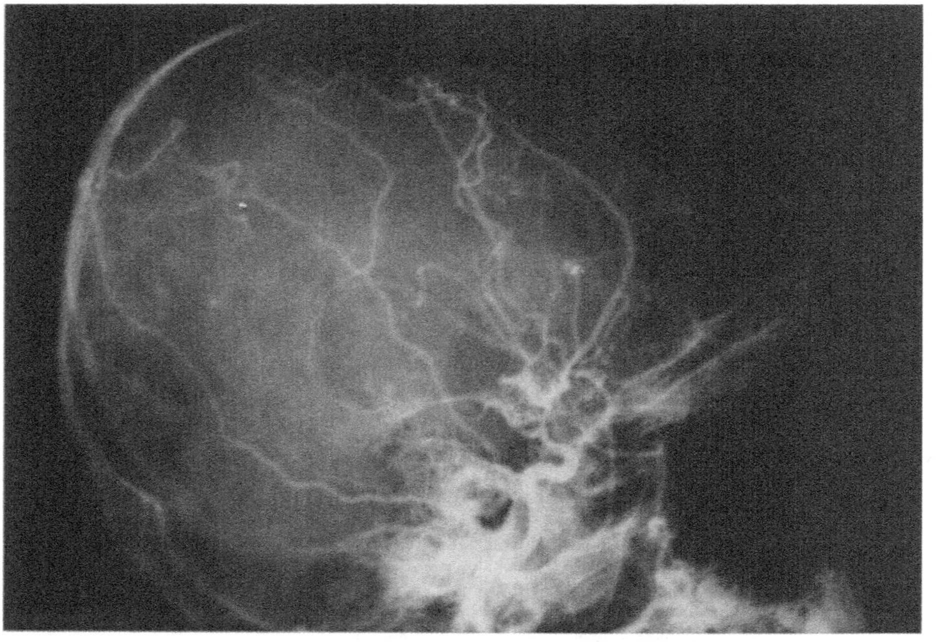

Fig. 145. Case 11: 10-year-old female. A case of quasi-moyamoya disease due to tuberculous vasculitis. Right carotid angiogram showed stenosis of the C_1 portion and moyamoya vessels in this region

12.7 Conclusion

In this chapter a variety of lesions which differ from the strict definition of true moyamoya disease have been discussed. These various forms of quasi-moyamoya disease are thought to provide us with a better understanding of true moyamoya disease.

By considering true moyamoya disease to be a lesion in which there is progressive stenosis and occlusion of the carotid fork bilaterally and, furthermore, in which the cause of the stenosis is not known, it seems most likely that true moyamoya disease is a special type of a generalized vascular disorder which has a strong predilection for developing at the bilateral terminal portion of the internal carotid arteries. Moreover, as discussed in an earlier chapter, the fact that vascular lesions similar to those seen at the terminal portion of the internal carotid artery and also found in many other organs in whole body autopsy studies strongly suggests that moyamoya disease is one manifestation of a general vascular disease.

Finally, the results of our experimental studies have gradually clarified that moyamoya disease is one manifestation of a generalized immune vascular disease in which the sympathetic nervous system, particularly the bilateral superior cervical ganglion (SCG), contributes to the development and/or aggravation of this disease.

References

1. Adams HP, Kassell NF, Wisoff HS, Drake CG (1979) Intracranial saccular aneurysm and moyamoya disease. Stroke 10: 174–179
2. Akai K, Hashimoto S, Moriyasu S (1967) On the net-like vascular anomaly on the cerebral artery. In: Kudo T (ed) A disease with abnormal intracranial vascular networks. Spontaneous occlusion of the cirle of Willis. Igaku shoin, Tokyo, pp 113–121
3. Aird RB (1959) Occipital and posterior electroencephalographic rhythms. Electroencephalogr Clin Neurophysiol 11: 637–656
4. Amine ARC, Moody RA, Meeks W (1977) Bilateral temporal-middle cerebral artery anastomosis or moymoya syndrome. Surg Neurol 8: 3–6
5. Ando K, Matsushima M, Yamamoto T, Suzuki Y, Yaga S, Oka H, Tsuji H (1967) Report of an autopsy case. In: Kudo T (ed) A disease with abnormal intracranial vascular networks. Spontaneous occlusion of the circle of Willis. Igaku shoin, Tokyo, pp 89–93
6. Angeline RM (1973) Multiple progressive intracranial arterial occlusions. Stroke 4: 380–386
7. Aoki N (1981) Two cases of pediatric moyamoya with intraventricular hemorrhage. In: Proceeding of the 10th Japanese conference on surgery of cerebral stroke. Neuron, Tokyo, pp 84–87
8. Aoki Y, Wada T, Hiraga H, Kodama N (1976) A case of cerebrovascular moyamoya disease. Clin Encephaloelectrogr (Osaka) 18: 522–523
9. Aoki Y, Kodama N, Hiraga H, Wada T (1977) Electroencephalographic findings in moyamoya disease. Brain Nerve (Tokyo) 29: 551–559
10. Arima H, Shimura M (eds) (1976) Advances of research for Kawasaki disease. Kindai Shuppan, Tokyo, pp 142–147 (in Japanese)
11. Arima M, Suda S, Namikawa M (1966) Infantile cases of progressive paralysis with teleangiectasis of basal ganglia and hypertension. Brain Nerve (Tokyo) 18: 549–551
12. Arimitsu T, Kikuchi H, Karasawa J, Shinomura T, Tsuchimoto S, Mitsugi T (1981) »Moyamoya« disease manifested with intracranial hemorrhage. In: Proceeding of the 10th Japanese conference on surgery of cerebral stroke. Neuron, Tokyo, pp 71–75
13. Arsemi C, Maretsis M, Horvath L (1971) Posttraumatic intracranial arterial spasm: Report of three cases. Acta Neurochir 24: 25–35
14. Asari S, Sato T, Sakurai M, Yamamoto Y, Sadamoto K (1981) Diagnosis of moyamoya disease by computed cerebral angiotomography. In: Proceeding of the 10th Japanese conference on surgery of cerebral stroke. Neuron, Tokyo, pp 113–118
15. Ausman JI, Moore J, Chou SN (1976) Spontaneous cerebral revascularization in a patient with STA-MCA anastomosis: Case report. J Neurosurg 44: 84–87
16. Beppu T, Arai Y, Kawamura H, Kitamura K, Kajita A (1971) Autopsy case of cerebral juxta-basal telangiectasia. Brain Nerve (Tokyo) 23: 1369–1380
17. Bingham WFB, Beguin EA, Ramirez-Lassepas (1980) Moyamoya disease in pregnancy. Wis Med J 79: 21–25
18. Boone SC, Sampson DS (1978) Observation on moyamoya disease: A case treated with superficial temporal-middle cerebral artery anastomosis. Surg Neurol 9: 189–193
19. Brodner RA (1981) An unusual moyamoya disease syndrome treated with superficial temporal-middle cerebral artery anastomosis: Case report. Milit Med 146: 52–54
20. Busch HFM (1969) Unusual collateral circulation in a child with cerebral arterial occlusion. Psychiatr Neurol Neurochir 72: 23–28
21. Carella A, Lamberti P, Perniola T, Livrea P, Federico F, Lochi L, Rosa AD, Fiore T, Liguori R (1977) Contributo clinico ed angiografico alla sindrome di moyamoya. Acta Neurol (Napoli) 32: 658–673
22. Carlson CB, Harvey FH, Loop J (1973) Progressive alternating hemiplegia in early childhood with basal arterial stenosis and telangiectasia: Moyamoya syndrome. Neurology 23: 734–744
23. Coakham HB, Duchen LW, Scaravilli F (1979) Moyamoya disease: Clinical and pathological report of a case with associated myopathy. J Neurol Neurosurg Psychiatry 42: 289–297

24. Cobb S (1931) The cerebral circulation: XIII The question of end-arteries of the brain an the mechanism of infarction. Arch Neurol Psychiatry 25: 273–280
25. Cochrane CG (1971) Mechanisms involved in the deposition of immune complexes in tissues. J Exp Med 134: 75–89
26. Cohen N, Berant M, Simon J (1980) Moyamoya and Fanconi's anemia. Pediatrics 65: 804–805
27. Crouzet G, Aguettaz G, Pellat J. Perret J, Barge M (1974) Les voies de supplèance au cours du Moyamoya. J Neuroradiol 1: 87–101
28. Debrun G, Lacour P (1974) A new case of moyamoya disease associated with several intracavernous aneurysms. Neuroradiology 7: 277–282
29. Dillon JD, Stokes H, Meirowsky AM (1975) Moyamoya disease. Surg Neurol 3: 233–236
30. Dixon FJ, Vasquez JJ, Weigle W, Cochrane CG (1958) The pathogenesis of serum sickness. Arch Pathol 65: 18–28
31. Dumas M, Girard PL, Collomb H (1972) Occlusions bilaterales de la carotide interne associee à une circulation de suppleance carotico-corticale, Transdurale, et du tipe moyamoya chez l'enfant noir. J Neurol Sci 16: 1–25
32. Dumas M, Girard PL, Konate S, N'Diaye IP (1973) Occlusions carotide sylviennes et Moya Moya chez l'enfant noir. Bull Soc Med Afr Noire Lang Fr 18: 67–71
33. Ebihara S, Gotoh F, Kanda T, Yamaguchi F, Nakahara K, Niimi T, Okayasu H (1977) Cerebral blood flow and metabolism in moyamoya disease. Acta Neurol Scand [Supple 64] 56: 404–405
34. Eguchi T, Oka H, Suzuki I, Mayanagi Y, Teraoka A (1981) Angiographical early venous filling, red cortical vein, intraarterial pressure and CBF values in moyamoya disease. In: Proceeding of the 10th Japanese conference on surgery of cerebral stroke. Neuron, Tokyo, pp 213–280
35. Ellison PH, Largent JA, Popp AJ (1981) Moya-moya disease associated with renal artery stenosis. Arch Neurol 38: 467
36. Endo H. Oikawa T. Yukawa H, Saiki I, Kanaya H (1981) Regional cerebral blood flow in patients with moyamoya disease. In: Proceeding of the 10th Japanese conference on surgery of cerebral stroke. Neuron, Tokyo, pp 179–183
37. Fisher CM (1959) Early-life carotid-artery occlusion associated with late intracranial hemorrhage. Lab Invest 8: 680–700
38. Floquet J (1975) Aspects anatomiques du syndrome moyamoya (Stenoses progressive des branches du polygone de willis). A propos de deux observations. Arch Anat Pathol 23: 151–158
39. Frackowiak RSJ, Lenzi GL, Jones T, Heather JD (1980) Quantitative measurement of regional cerebral blood flow and oxygen metabolism in man using ^{15}O and positron emission tomography. Theory, procedure and normal values. J Comput Assist Tomogr 4: 727–736
40. Fujiwara S, Kodama N, Sakurai Y, Hori S (1978) CT scan in moyamoya disease of children. Brain Dev 10: 446–451
41. Fujiwara S, Yonemitsu T, Kasai N, Kodama N, Suzuki J (1981) Transdural anastomosis in moyamoya disease — vault moyamoya. In: Proceeding of the 10th Japanese conference on surgery of cerebral stroke. Neuron, Tokyo, pp 129–133
42. Fukada T, Ishizaki F (1978) A case of moyamoya disease with cavum septi pellucidi. Neurol Med (Tokyo) 9: 95
43. Fukai H, Satoh S, Ueki Y (1966) Study of the diseases showing the abnormal vascular network at the base of the brain. Brain Nerve (Tokyo) 18: 519–525
44. Fukawa O, Aihara M, Ishii K, Kikuchi J, Mashiyama S, Katayama M, Kogure T (1981) Middle cerebral artery occlusion with moyamoya phenomenon. First report: Clinical course and angiographical findings. In: Proceeding of the 10th Japanese conference on surgery of cerebral stroke. Neuron, Tokyo, pp 36–41
45. Fukuzawa J, Kutsuzawa T (1978) An autopsy case showing so-called moyamoya vessels. In: Reports by the research committee on spontaneous occlusion of the circle of Willis. Japanese Ministry of Health and Welfare, Tokyo, pp 91–102
46. Fukuyama Y, Suzuki Y, Segawa A (1965) Acute repeated transient hemiplegia in child. Brain Nerve (Tokyo) 17: 757–760

47. Galligioni F, Andrioli GC, Marin G, Briani S, Iraci G (1971) Hypoplasia of the internal carotid artery associated with cerebral pseudoangiomatosis: Report of 4 cases. AJR 112: 251–262
48. Gemende G, Kagel KO (1978) Beitrag zum Moyamoya-Syndrome. Zentralbl Neurochir 39: 301–310
49. Gerlach J, Jensen HP, Koos W, Krans H (eds) (1967) Pädiatrische Neurochirurgie. Thieme, Stuttgart
50. Gibbs FA, Gibbs EL (eds) (1952) Atlas of electroencephalography, vol II. Addison-Wesley, Cambridge
51. Goto F, Ebihara S, Koto A, Nakahara K, Niimi T (1978) Cerebral blood flow and metabolisms in occlusion of the circle of Willis. In: Reports by the research committee on spontaneous occlusion of the circle of Willis. Japanese Ministry of Health and Welfare, Tokyo, pp 81–86
52. Goto, F. Ebihara S, Nakahara K, Niimi T (1979) Cerebral blood flow and metabolisms in occlusion of the circle of Willis. In: Reports by the research committee on spontaneous occlusion of the circle of Willis. Japanese Ministry of Health and Welfare, Tokyo, pp 83–87
53. Goto F, Ebihara S, Sakai F, Kitagawa Y (1980) Cerebral blood flow and metabolisms in occlusion of the circle of Willis. In: Reports by the research committee on spontaneous occlusion of the circle of Willis. Japanese Ministry of Health and Welfare, Tokyo, pp 65–71
54. Goto F, Ebihara S, Sakai F, Kitagawa Y (1981) Cerebral blood flow and metabolisms in occlusion of the circle of Willis. In: Reports by the research committee on spontaneous occlusion of the circle of Willis. Japanese of Health and Welfare, Tokyo, pp 65–96
55. Goto F, Ebihara S, Takagi Y, Kitagawa Y, Hata T (1982) Cerebral blood flow and metabolisms in occlusion of the circle of Willis. In: Reports by the research committee on spontaneous occlusion of the circle of Willis. Japanese Ministry of Health and Welfare, Tokyo, pp 90–97
56. Goto Y (1970) An autopsy case showing abnormal intracranial vascular networks. Clin Neurol (Tokyo) 10: 420
57. Gradzki J, Wroblewski T (1980) Zespol moyamoya. Pol Przeg Radiol Med Nukl 4: 273–277
58. Gutierrez-Mahoney CG, Schechter MM (1972) The myth of the rete mirabile in man. Neuroradiology 4: 141–158
59. Halonen H (1973) Occlusive disease of intracranial main arteries with collateral networks in children. Neuropediatrie 4: 187–206
60. Handa H, Tani E, Handa J, Kondo A, Kikuchi H, Sato K (1967) Idiopathic occlusive arterial disorders in the cervical region and the main trunks of the cerebral arteries in Japan. In: Kudo T (ed) A disease with abnormal intracranial vascular networks. Spontaneous occlusion of the circle of Willis. Igaku shoin, Tokyo, pp 83–88
61. Handa H, Tani E, Kajikawa H, Satoh K, Yamashita J, Osaka K, Haebara H, Tamegai M, Kyogoku M (1969), Clinicopathological study on an adult case with cerebral arterial rete. Brain Nerve (Tokyo) 21: 181–191
62. Handa J, Handa H (1972) Progressive cerebral arterial occlusive disease: Analysis of 27 cases. Neuroradiology 3: 119–133
63. Handa J, Matsuda I, Handa H, Nakano Y, Komuro H, Okuno T, Aii H (1977) Computed tomography in »Moya-moya«: Summary of 16 cases. Brain Nerve (Tokyo) 29: 1067–1074
64. Handa J, Nakano Y, Okuno T, Komuro H, Hohjyo H, Handa H (1977) Computerized tomography in moyamoya syndrome. Surg Neurol (Tokyo) 7: 315–319
65. Hara K, Nishi T, Yuasa R, Fujimoto J (1966) Study of the cases showing the abnormal vascular network at the base of the brain. Brain Nerve (Tokyo) 18: 527–531
66. Hashimoto T (1970) A case showing the abnormal vascular network at the base of brain with hypoplasia of unilateral renal artery. Saishinigaku (Osaka) 25: 916–921 (in Japanese)
67. Hayasaki K (1970) A case of schizophrenic state combined with intracranial rete mirabile vascularity. Brain Nerve (Tokyo) 22: 1319–1323
68. Hayashi N, Takeuchi T, Sugawara T, Gotoh T, Tsubokawa T, Moriyasu N (1975) Cerebral circulation of the OWN disease (so-called »Moyamoya« disease). Blood Vessel (Tokyo) 6: 956–964
69. Heiss WD, Horcajada J, Reisner T (1973) Regionale Störungen der Hirndurchblutung bei Moyamoya-Erkrankung. ROFO 119: 223–230

70. Henschen C (1950) Operative revascularization des zirkulatorisch geschädigten Gehirns durch Anlegen gestielter Muskellappen. Encephalo-Myo-Synangiose. Langenbecks Arch Klin Chir 264: 392–401
71. Higashi K, Hatano M, Maza T (1974) Disease with abnormal intracranial vascular network complicated with intracerebral haematoma. J Neurol Neurosurg Psychiatry 37: 365–369
72. Hilar SK, et al. (1971) Primary cerebral arterial occlusive disease in children. Part II: Neurocutaneous syndromes. Radiology 99: 87–94
73. Hinshaw DB, Thompson JR, Hasso AN (1976) Adult arteriosclerotic moyamoya. Radiology 118: 633–636
74. Hiraga H, Aoki Y, Kodama N (1980) Electroencephalographic findings in moyamoya disease: its diagnostic value and classification. Clin Encephaloelectrogr (Osaka) 22 (8): 513–526
75. Hirano M, Sakurai S (1972) Psychiatric symptoms and signs associated with spontaneous occlusion of the circle of Willis. A case report and studies of 379 cases in Japan. Psychiatr Med (Tokyo) 14: 329–338
76. Hirayama A, Kowada M, Fukasawa H, Itoh Z, Matsuoka S, Gitoh Y (1974) Cerebrovascular moyamoya disease — a case report and review of 12 autopsy cases in Japan. Brain Nerve (Tokyo) 26: 1215–1225
77. Hoare M, Keogh AJ (1974) Cerebrovascular moyamoya disease. Br Med J 1: 430–432
78. Hojo K, Kobayashi Y, Kawakita Y (1967) Juvenile bilateral carotid artery occlusion, a histopathologic study of the vascular change. In: Kudo T (ed) A disease with abnormal intracranial vascular networks. Spontaneous occlusion of the circle of Willis. Igaku shoin, Tokyo, pp 104–113
79. Honma A, Tsutsui T, Sunami T, Endo H, Nagao S, Doi A, Nishimoto S (1981) Electrolic-physiology of Moyamoya disease. In: Reports by the research committee on spontaneous occlusion of the circle of Willis. Japanese Ministry of Health and Welfare, Tokyo, pp 35–44
80. Hori T, Fukushima T, Tsuchida T, Ishijima B, Manaka S, Hirakawa K (1971) A case of cerebral juxta-basal telangiectasia with intracerebral hematoma. Brain Nerve (Tokyo) 23: 1403–1408
81. Hosoda Y (1974) A pathomorphological analysis of so-called »Spontaneous occlusion of the circle of Willis« (Cerebrovascular »Moyamoya disease«). Brain Nerve (Tokyo) 26: 471–481
82. Hosoda Y (1974) A pathological study of so-called »Spontaneous occlusion of the circle of Willis« (cerebrovascular »Moyamoya« disease) with a special reference to resions of the proximal region of occluded arteries. J College Angiology (Tokyo) 14: 119–127
83. Hosoda Y (1975) Pathology of so-called »Spontaneous occlusion of the circle of Willis« (Cerebrovascular »Moyamoya« disease). Blood Vessel (Tokyo) 6: 946–955
84. Hosoda Y, Ishii Y (1978) Pathological study about arterial region in two autopsy cases of disease of occlusion of the circle of Willis. In: Reports by the research committee on spontaneous occlusion of the circle of Willis. Japanese Ministry of Health and Welfare, Tokyo, pp 108–115
85. Hosoda Y, Ishii Y, Mukai M, Yamada T, Tekigi T, Nomura M, Otsuka K, Abe H, Tsuru M, Murase H (1979) Pathological study about three autopsy cases showing abnormal vascular net-work. In: Reports by the research committee on spontaneous occlusion of the circle of Willis. Japanese Ministry of Health and Welfare, Tokyo, pp 116–131
86. Hosoda Y, Ishii Y, Mukai M, Sakuma K, Furukawa T, Fukuda S, Yamada F, Murase I, Kasahara M (1981) Pathological changes of cerebrum and cerebral vessels in disease of occlusion of the circle of Willis. In: Reports by the research committee on spontaneous occlusion of the circle of Willis. Japanese Ministry of Health and Welfare, Tokyo, pp 139–147
87. Houser OW, Baker HL, Sandock BA, Holley KE (1971 Cepharic arteriol fibromascular dysplasia. Radiology 101: 605–611
88. Ichijo S (1977) Fourteen and six Hz positive spikes in a patient of »Moyamoya disease«. Clin Encephaloelectrogr (Osaka) 19: 145
89. Iivanainen M, Vuolio M, Halonen V (1973) Occlusive disease of intracranial main arteries with collateral networks (moyamoya disease) in adults. Acta Neurol Scand 49: 307–322

90. Imaizumi M, Nukada S, Yoneda S, Takano T, Hasegawa K, Abe H (11978) Tuberous sclerosis with moyamoya disease: Case report. Med J Osaka Univ 28: 345–353
91. Iraci G, Marin G, Andrioli G, Feltrin G (1972) Further observation on the so-called »Japanese cerebrovascular disease«. AJR 115: 35–38
92. Ishikawa M, Handa H, Mori K, Matsudo I (1979) Moyamoya vessels on the tumor in the sellar region. Arch Jpn Chir 48: 639–644
93. Isono M, Yonemitsu T, Fujiwara S, Kodama N, Suzuki J (1981) Epidemiological study on moyamoya disease: From the experiences of 100 cases. In: Proceeding of the 10th Japanese conference on surgery of cerebral stroke. Neuron, Tokyo, pp 3–7
94. Itoh T, Kubo K, Kawamoto M (1967) Some references to 3 cases with abnormal vascular network in the cerebral basal region. Brain Nerve (Tokyo) 19:37–43
95. Iwata K (1967) Clinical experience on intracranial peculiar rete mirable vascularity with acute stenosis of distal end of the internal carotid arteries. In: Kudo T (ed) A disease with abnormal intracranial vascular networks. Spontaneous occlusion of the circle of Willis. Igaku shoin, Tokyo, pp 53–56
96. Izawa M, Sentoh S (1981) A case of cerebrovascular moyamoya disease associated with basilar aneurysm. Neurol Surg (Tokyo) 9: 365–370
97. Kamio M, Shimizu H, Yabuuchi H (1980) Clinical and electroencephalographic features of cerebrovascular diseases in children. Clin Encephaloelectrogr (Osaka) 22: 537–546
98. Kamisaka A, Hiratsuka H, Inaba Y (1972) A case of an aneurysm arising in abnormal intracranial vascular networks. Brain Nerve (Tokyo) 24: 464–468
99. Kanaya H, Ishikawa Y, Osawa K, Nemoto T, Ono S, Kumagai O, Horie Y, Oana K (1976) Our consideration concerning the origin of cerebrobasal arterial rate. In: Kudo T (ed) A disease with abnormal intracranial vascular networks. Spontaneous occlusion of the circle of Willis. Igaku shoin, Tokyo, pp 43–45
100. Kanayama S, Niizuma H (1981) Cerebrovascular moyamoya disease: Study of collateral circulation with microangiography and translucidation. In: Proceeding of the 10th Japanese conference on surgery of cerebral stroke. Neuron, Tokyo, pp 154–157
101. Kaneko H, Ishizaki T, Itoh G, Makifuchi T (1969) An autopsy case of »Rete mirable« at the cerebral base. J Niigata Med Soc (Niigata) 83: 725–727
102. Kaneko H, Okamura A, Nishida K, Watanabe M (1971) An autopsy case of intracranial rete mirable. Brain Nerve (Tokyo) 23: 1381–1387
103. Kaneko H, Okamura A, Obata N (1971) An autopsy case of the occlusion of Willis' circle with idiopathic cardiomegalia. J Niigata Med Soc (Niigata) 85: 534–538
104. Kaplan AH, Ford HD (1966) The brain vascular system. Elsevier, New York
105. Kaplan HA (1965) The lateral perforating branches of the anterior and middle cerebral arteries. J Neurosurg 23: 305–310
106. Karasawa J, Kikuchi H, Furuse S (1977) A surgical treatment of »Moyamoya« disease »encephalo-myo synagiosis«. Neurol Med Chir (Tokyo) 17 (I): 30–37
107. Karasawa J, Kikuchi H, Furuse K, Sakaki J, Yoshida Y, Onishi H, Sugiyama T, Hamamoto Y (1977) Clinical signs and treatment of »moyamoya« disease. — Study of seven children —. Pedriatr Clin (Tokyo) 30: 86–92
108. Karasawa J, Kikuchi H, Furuse S, Kawamura J, Sasaki T (1978) Treatment of moyamoya disease with STA-MCA anastomosis. J Neurosurg 49: 679–688
109. Karasawa J, Kikuchi H, Kawamura J, Sakai T (1980) Intracranial transplantation of the omentum for cerebrovascular moyamoya disease: A two-year follow-up study. Surg Neurol 14: 444–449
110. Karasawa J, Kikuchi H, Furuse S, Itoh K, Takahashi N, Sakashita Y, Kamata K (1980) Computed tomography in »Moyamoya« disease: Pre- and postoperative findings. Prog Comput Tomogr (Osaka) 2: 311–317
111. Karasawa J, Kikuchi H, Takahashi N, Utsumi S, Iwayama K, Yamamoto J (1980) Electroencephalographic study of »Moyamoya« disease in children: — pre and post — surgical EEG's changes and its pathophysiology —. Clin Encephaloelectrogr (Osaka) 22: 527–536
112. Karasawa J, Kikuchi H, Matsumoto A, Ito K, Takahashi N (1981) Surgical treatment of »Moyamoya« disease: Follow-up study during 3.5 years and over. In: Proceeding of the 10th Japanese conference on surgery of cerebral stroke. Neuron, Tokyo, pp 306–312

113. Karasawa J, Kikuchi H, Kuriyama Y, Sawa T, Kuro M, Kobayashi K, Koike T, Mitsugi T (1981) Cerebral hemodynamics in »Moyamoya« disease. — II. Measurements of cerebral circulation and metabolism by use of the argon desaturation method in pre- and post-neurosurgical procedures. Neurol Med Chir (Tokyo) 21: 1161–1168
114. Kasai N, Fujiwara S, Kodama N, Suzuki J (1981) Surgical treatment in moyamoya disease. In: Proceeding of the 10th Japanese conference on surgery of cerebral stroke. Neuron, Tokyo, pp 221–224
115. Kasai N, Fujiwara S, Kodama N, Yonemitsu T, Suzuki J (1982) The experimental study on causal genesis of Moyamoya disease — Correlation with immunological reaction and sympathetic nerve influence for vascular changes — Neurol Surg (Tokyo) 10: 251–261
116. Katoh H, Nara M, Sakurai Y (1973) A case of moyamoya disease showing abnormal EEG by hyperventilation. Clin Encephaloelectrogr (Osaka) 15: 326
117. Katoh Y, Katada K, Shinomiya Y, Sano H, Kanno T (1981) Verification of surgical cases of occlusion of circle of Willis. In: Proceeding of the 10th Japanese conference on surgery of cerebral stroke. Neuron, Tokyo, pp 291–296
118. Katsuki S, Tomonaga H (1961) Constructive characteristics of cerebral blood vessels — Study using injection of synthetic rubber —. Adv Neurol Sci (Tokyo) 5: 277–289
119. Kawabuchi J (1967) Teleangiectatic malformation of bilateral internal carotid artery. In: Kudo T (ed) A disease with abnormal intracranial vascular networks. Spontaneous occlusion of the circle of Willis. Igaku shin, Tokyo, pp 46–47
120. Kawakita Y, Abe K (1965) Spontaneous thrombosis of the internal carotid artery in children. Folia Psychiatr Neurol Jpn 19: 245–255
121. Kikuchi H, Karasawa J (1976) Extra-intracranial arterial anastomosis in ten patients with moyamoya syndrome. In: Schmiedek P (ed) Microsurgery for stroke. Springer, Berlin Heidelberg New York, pp 260–263
122. Kinoshita J (1971) An autopsy case of spontaneous occlusion of the circle of Willis. Adv Neurol Sci (Tokyo) 15: 780
123. Kitahara T, Ariga N, Yamaura A, Makino H, Maki Y (1979) Familial occurrence of moyamoya disease: report of three Japanese families. J Neurol Neurosurg Psychiatry 42: 208–214
124. Kitahara T, Senba A, Yamaura A, Makino H, Okumura K (1981) Genetical and immunological analysis on moyamoya disease. In: Proceeding of the 10th Japanese conference on surgery of cerebral stroke. Neuron, Tokyo, pp 27–30
125. Kitamura K, Kinoshita K (1967) Angiographic evidence of collateral circulation of the brain. in: Kudo T (ed) A disease with abnormal intracranial vascular networks. Spontaneous occlusion of the circle of Willis. Igaku shoin, Tokyo, pp 38–41
126. Klaus E, Fárková H, Urbánek K (1970) Ein Fall von »Moyamoya Disease« (Nishimoto-Takeuchi-Kudo-Syndrome). Fortschr Geb Roentgenstr Nuklearmed 113: 603–608
127. Kobayashi S, Tazaki Y, Kanda T, Koga H (1980) Systemic angitis associated with abnormal rete mirabile and occlusion of the bilateral carotid arteries: an autopsy case. Jpn J Stroke (Tokyo) 2: 42–48
128. Kobayashi K, Takeuchi S, Tsuchida T, Itoh J (1981) Encephalo-myo-synangiosis in moyamoya disease: With special reference to postoperative angiography. Neurol Med Chir (Tokyo) 21: 1229–1238
129. Kodama N (1971) The study on the aging of the perforating branches and its possibility of collateral pathway: concerning cerebrovascular »Moyamoya« disease. Brain Nerve (Tokyo) 23: 1389–1402
130. Kodama N, Suzuki J (1975) Cerebrovascular moyamoya disease IIIrd report — The study on the aging of the perforating branches and the possibility of collateral pathway. Neurol Med Chir (Tokyo) 15 (I): 55–67
131. Kodama N, Suzuki J (1978) Moyamoya disease associated with aneurysm. J Neurosurg 48: 565–569
132. Kodama N, Mineura K, Suzuki J, Kitaoka T, Kurashima Y, Takahashi S (1976) Cerebrovascular moyamoya disease associated with aneurysm at the peripheral portion of the posterior chorioidal artery. Neurol Surg (Tokyo) 4: 985–991
133. Kodama N, Mineura K, Suzuki J, Onuma T (1976) Ventricular hemorrhage due to chronic cerebral ischemia. Brain Nerve (Tokyo) 28: 823–831

134. Kodama N, Mineura K, Suzuki J (1977) Cerebrovascular moyamoya disease associated with basilar aneurysm. Neurol Surg (Tokyo) 5: 65–69
135. Kodama N, Aoki Y, Hiraga H, Wada T, Suzuki J (1979) Electroencephalographic findings in children with moyamoya disease. Arch Neurol 36: 16–19
136. Kodama N, Fujiwara S, Horie Y, Kayama T, Suzuki J (1980) Transdural anastomosis in moyamoya disease: vault moyamoya. Neurol Surg (Tokyo) 8: 729–737
137. Kodama N, Fujiwara S, Kasai N, Yonemitsu T, Suzuki J (1981) The experimental study on causal genesis of moyamoya disease: correlation with immunological reaction and sympathetic nerve influence for vascular changes. In: Proceeding of the 10th Japanese conference on surgery of cerebral stroke. Neuron, Tokyo, pp 17–26
138. Koike T, Kikuchi H, Karasawa J, Kobayashi K, Arimitsu T, Mitsugi T, Kuriyama Y, Kozuka T, Nishimura T (1981) Evaluation of radioisotope studies after surgical treatment in »Moyamoya« disease. In: Proceeding of the 10th Japanese conference on surgery of cerebral stroke. Neuron, Tokyo, pp 318–322
139. Kowada M, Monma F, Kikuchi K (1979) Intracranial aneurysm associated with cerebrovascular moyamoya disease: report of a case and review of 13 cases. Br J Radiol 52: 236–237
140. Krayenbühl HA, Yasargil MG (1965) Cerebral angiography. Butterworth, London
141. Krayenbühl HA (1975) The moyamoya syndrome and neurosurgeon. Surg Neurol 4: 353–360
142. Kudo T (1965) Personal opinion for disease with abnormal intracranial vascular networks. Brain Nerve (Tokyo) 17: 37–38
143. Kudo T (1965) Juvenile occlusion of the circle of Willis. Clin Neurol (Tokyo) 5: 607–627
144. Kudo T (1966) Resemble case of spontaneous occlusion of the circle of Willis. Clin Neurol (Tokyo) 6: 336–347
145. Kudo T (1966) A disease of spontaneous occlusion of the circle of Willis. Brain Nerve (Tokyo) 18: 889–896
146. Kudo T (1967) A disease with abnormal intracranial vascular network. Spontaneous occlusion of the circle of Willis. Igaku shoin, Tokyo
147. Kudo T (1968) Spontaneous occlusion of the circle of Willis. Neurology 18: 485–496
148. Kudo T (1971) A disease of spontaneous occlusion of the circle of Willis. Moyamoya disease. Medicine 28: 465–469 [in Japanese]
149. Kudo T (1978) A disease of spontaneous occlusion of the circle of Willis. Moyamoya disease. Adv Neurol Sci (Tokyo) 22: 808–809
150. Kudo T, Takayama R, Mikawakuchi K, Ishimori S, Otake S, Nakagawa K (1957) Occlusion of internal carotid artery. Brain Nerve (Tokyo) 9: 757
151. Kudo T, Handa H, Kuwabara T, Suzuki J, Hosoda Y, Nishimoto S (1971) A disease with abnormal intracranial vascular networks. Transactions of the 18th general assembly of Japan medical congress, Tokyo, pp 1253–1273
152. Kuro M, Karasawa J, Kuriyama T, Kikuchi H (1981) Anesthetic management of »Moyamoya« disease in children. In: Proceeding of the 10th Japanese conference on surgery of cerebral stroke. Neuron, Tokyo, pp 207–211
153. Kuromaru S (1963) Juvenile case showing abnormal rete angiomatous appearance on cerebral angiography. In: Proceedings of the IIIrd meeting of clinical neurology in children.
154. Kurt HHM (1978) Cerebrovascular disease in sickle cell anemia. Clinical, pathological and radiological correlations. Stroke 9: 45–52
155. Kyogoku K, Kubota A, Nose M, Watanabe S, Ukai K, Matsumoto M, Shimomura R, Shirane H, Kizaki T (1975) Pathological changes of vessels by immune complex. Jpn J Clin Med (Osaka) 33: 2746–2761
156. Kyogoku K, Oguma S, Yaginuma N, Sawai T, Kawashima M, Nagao K (1980) Reports by the research committee on an incurable disease. Japanese Ministry of Health and Welfare, Tokyo, pp 49–55
157. Lamas E, Diez Lobato R, Cabello A, Abad JM (1978) Multiple intracranial arterial occlusions (moyamoya disease) in patients with neurofibromatosis: one case report with sutopsy. Acta Neurochir 45: 133–145

158. Lanzi G, Bianchi E, Pezzotta S, Cornalba G (1974) La malattia di moyamoya: Illustrazione di un caso. Minerva Pediatr 26: 1958–1968
159. Lee MLK, Cheung EMT (1973) Moyamoya disease as a cause of subarachnoid haemorrhage in chinese. Brain 96: 623–628
160. Leeds NE, Abbott KH (1965) Collateral circulation in cerebrovascular disease in childhood via rete mirabile and perforating branches of anterior choroidal and posterior cerebral arteries. Radiology 85: 628–634
161. Lehmann G, Vincentelli F, Ebagosti A (1980) Anomalies rares du polygone de willis: Re trajet infra-optique des artéres cérébrales antérieures. Neurochirurgie 26: 243–246
162. Le Marec B, Herry JF, Signargout J, Guy G, Faivre J, Simon J, Sénécal J (1973) Le moyamoya ou maladie de nishimoto: A propos de trois cas. Pédiatrie 28: 133–148
163. Levesque M, Bories J, Lefebvre J (1973) Moyamoya: A propos de six observations. Ann Radiol (Paris) 16: 27–40
164. Likavcan M, Benko J, Papiernikovä E, Lindtnerová L (1979) »Moyamoya« syndrom s hyperlipoproteinemiou. Typ IIa. Desk Neurol Neurochir 42: 49–53
165. Mabuchi A, Tanabe H, Fujikawa Y, Fujimoto K, Nakata K (1973) An autopsy case of the abnormal network of the intracranial artery: congenital dysplagia of the cerebral artery. Brain Nerve (Tokyo) 25: 1759–1765
166. Maeda T, Mori H, Hisada K, Sugino M (1979) Radionuclide cerebral angiography in moyamoya disease. Clin Nucl Med 4: 513–515
167. Maki Y, Nakada Y (1965) Autopsy cases showing angiomatous anomaly of carotid artery at the base of the brain. Brain Nerve (Tokyo) 17: 764–766
168. Maki Y, Horie T, Nakada Y (1967) A report of the autopsied case. In: Kudo T (ed) A disease with abnormal intracranial vascular networks. Spontaneous occlusion of the circle of Willis. Igaku shoin, Tokyo, pp 98–101
169. Maki Y, Nakada Y, Nose T, Yoshii Y (1976) Clinical and radioisotopic follow-up study of »moyamoya«. Childs Brain 2: 257–271
170. Maki Y, Nose T, Tanoue K, Abe T (1981) Platelet aggregation in patients with moyamoya disease. Angiology 32: 522–528
171. Mathew NT, Abraham J, Chandy J (1970) Cerebral angiographic features in tuberculous meningitis. Neurology 20: 1015–1023
172. Matsuo K, Shiraishi M, Takebayashi S, Muraki M, Kaneko (1981) Ultrastructural aspects of cerebral arteries in moyamoya disease — particulary with respect to perforating arteries and cerebral hemorrhage —. In: Proceeding of the 10th Japanese conference on surgery of cerebral stroke. Neuron, Tokyo, pp 147–153
173. Matsushima Y, Fukai N, Tanaka K, Tsuruoka S, Inaba Y, Aoyagi M, Ohno K (1981) A new surgical treatment of moyamoya disease in children: a preliminary report. Surg Neurol 15: 313–320
174. Matsushima Y, Fukai N, Aoyagi M, Tanaka K, Takasato Y, Inaba Y (1981) Indication of encephalo-duro-arterio-synangiosis to adult moyamoya patients. In: Proceeding of the 10th Japanese conference on surgery of cerebral stroke. Neuron, Tokyo, pp 225–229
175. Mauro AJ, Johnson ES, Chikos PM, Alvord EC (1980) Lipohyalinosis and miliary microaneurysms causing cerebral hemorrhage in a patient with moyamoya. Stroke 11: 405–412
176. Meriwether RP, Barnett HG, Echols DH (1976) Moyamoya disease as a cause of subarachnoid hemorrhage in a Negro patient. Case report. J Neurosurg 44: 620–622
177. Minguetti G, Ferreira MVC (1981) Moyamoya disease. CT scan study of a Brazilian-born Japanese girl. Neuro-Psiquiatria (São Paulo) 39: 101–105
178. Mitsumoto T, Kikuchi H, Karasawa J, Koike T, Kuriyama Y, Sawada T, Kuro M (1981) Evaluation of CBF studies, changes of CBF and cerebral metabolism after surgical treatment in »Moyamoya« disease. In: Proceeding of the 10th Japanese conference on surgery of cerebral stroke. Neuron, Tokyo, pp 323–327
179. Miyasaka K, Takei H, Nakagawa T, Abe H, Tsuru M (1978) A disease showing »Moyamoya« vascular network in base of brain: evaluation of angiography and cranial computed tomography. Brain Nerve (Tokyo) 20: 1083–1091
180. Mizukawa N (1975) Moyamoya disease — its symptoms and etiology. Blood Vessel (Tokyo) 6: 937–945

181. Mizukawa N, Ueda K, Takeuchi S, Nishimoto S (1974) Abnormal vascular networks at the base of the brain: Statistical study and its problem. Igakuno Ayumi (Tokyo) 91: 279
182. Moene Y, Taillandier P, Revol M, Courjon J (1973) Étude deś modifications EEG dans le syndrome Moya-Moya. Rev Electroencephalogr Europhysiol 4: 304–307
183. Momma F, Kowada M, Kikuchi A, Kogo U (1979) Cerebrovascular Moyamoya disease associated with basilar artery aneurysm. Report of a case. Clin Radiol (Tokyo) 24: 285–288
184. Moriyasu N, Nishio S (1965) Five cases of network like vascular anomaly of internal carotid artery. Brain Nerve (Tokyo) 17: 761–763
185. Mount LA, Taveras JM (1957) Arteriographic demonstration of the collateral circulation of the cerebral hemispheres. Arch Neurol Psychiatry 78: 235–253
186. Mracek Z, Kohoutek V (1974) Syndrom moyamoya. Cab Le Desk 113: 1561–1565
187. Murakami M, Iijima S, Takeo H, Morita K, Amaki I, Uchida T, Kobayashi M, Sakurai I (1979) A case of polyarteritis nudosa which initially indicated neurological symptoms. Clin Neurol (Tokyo) 11: 39–44
188. Murphy M (1980) Progressive vascular changes in moyamoya syndrome. Stroke 11: 656–658
189. Nagai H, Shibata T, Nitta M, Umemura K, Takagi A, Iwayama K (1981) Cerebral hemodynamics in spontaneous occlusion of the circle of Willis. In: Reports by the research committee on spontaneous occlusion of the circle of Willis. Japanese Ministry of Health and Welfare, Tokyo, pp 65–70
190. Nagai H, Shibata T, Iwayama K (1982) Cerebral hemodynamics in spontaneous occlusion of the circle of Willis. Part II. In: Reports by the research committee on spontaneous occlusion of the circle of Willis. Japanese Ministry of Health and Welfare, Tokyo, pp 105–110
191. Nagamine Y, Sonobe M, Takahashi S (1980) Multiple aneurysms associated with moyamoya disease. Neurol Surg (Tokyo) 8: 275–282
192. Nagamine Y, Takahashi S, Sonobe M (1981) Multiple intracranial aneurysms associated with moyamoya disease. Case report. J Neurosurg 54: 673–676
193. Nagamine Y, Kasai N, Fujiwara S, Kodama N, Suzuki J, Fukasawa H (1981) Pathological study of 10 autopsy cases on moyamoya diseases. In: Proceedings of the 10th Japanese conference on surgery of cerebral stroke. Neuron, Tokyo, pp 141–146
194. Nagase K (1958) Histopathological pictures, innervation and clinical considerations of human palatine tonsils. J Oto-Rhino-Laryngol Soc Jpn (Tokyo) 61: 1481–1488
195. Nagaya T, Nukui H, Miyagi O, Tamada J, Kawabuchi J (1981) Cerebral hemodynamics in cases with moyamoya disease. In: Proceeding of the 10th Japanese conference on surgery of cerebral stroke. Neuron, Tokyo, pp 174–178
196. Nakada Y, Yoshii Y, Nose T, Tomono Y, Maki Y, Horie T (1978) Follow-up study of moyamoya in adult patients. Neurol Med Chir (Tokyo) 18: 75–82
197. Nakagawa Y, Shimoyama M, Kashiwaba T, Suzuki Y, Goto S, Miyasaka K, Takei H, Goto S, Ohtsuka K, Abe H, Tsuru M (1981) Reconstructive operation of moyamoya diseases and its problems. Surg Neurol 9: 305–314
198. Nakagawa Y, Kinomoto H, Akino M, Horikawa D, Tsuru M, Ito K, Sugimoto S, Takei H, Nishiya M, Tokuda S, Sato M (1981) Significance of basal moyamoya vessels on cerebral circulation in moyamoya disease. In: Proceeding of the 10th Japanese conference on surgery of cerebral stroke. Neuron, Tokyo, pp 184–188
199. Nakagawa Y, Ikoda T, Ohtsuka K, Abe T, Tsuru M, Takei H, Sugimoto S, Goto S, Shimoyama M, Suzuki Y (1981) Indication of reconstructive operation for moyamoya disease and ideal operative methods. In: Proceeding of the 10th Japanese conference on surgery of cerebral stroke. Neuron, Tokyo, pp 230–235
200. Nakagawa K, Fujishima M, Numaguchi Y, Omae T (1979) Thalamic hemorrhage in moyamoya disease. A case report. Angiology 30: 856–860
201. Narumi S, Nishimura K, Fuchizawa K, Hidaka T (1976) Three cases of the moyamoya disease found in an inbred family. Brain Nerve (Tokyo) 28: 1201–1205
202. Nishijima M, Sakurai Y, Onuma T, Elbina T, Suzuki J (1978) Surgical treatment of thalamic hermorrhage. In: Proceeding of the 7th Japanese conference on surgery of cerebral stroke. Neuron, Tokyo, pp 100–103

203. Nishimoto A (1976) Angiographic criteria of the cerebrovascular Moyamoya disease. Adv Neurol Sci (Tokyo) 20: 758–767
204. Nishimoto A (1976) Moyamoya disease: a disease with abnormal vascular networks at the base of the brain. In: Current encyclopedia of surgery (suppl 1976–B). Nakayama shoten, Tokyo, pp 125–139
205. Nishimoto A (1978) Epidemiology and etiology of Moyamoya disease. Jpn J Clin Med (Tokyo) 36: 614–620
207. Nishimoto A, Mizukawa N (1975) So-called »moyamoya disease« from the neurosurgical standpoints. Neuro Med (Tokyo) 3: 37–45
208. Nishimoto A, Oube H (1980) Summary of clinical survey. In: Reports by the research committee on spontaneous occlusion of the circle of Willis. Japanese Ministry of Health and Welfare, Tokyo, pp 99–105
209. Nishimoto A, Sugio R (1964) Hemangiomatous malformation of bilateal internal carotid artery at the base of brain. In: Proceedings of the 6th Annual Meeting of the Neuro-Radiological Association of Japan pp 2–9
210. Nishimoto A, Takeuchi S (1967) Cerebral basal rete mirabile. In: Kudo T (ed) A disease with abnormal intracranial vascular networks. Spontaneous occlusion of the circle of Willis. Igaku shoin, Tokyo, pp 56–59 [in Japanese]
211. Nishimoto A, Takeuchi S (1968) Abnormal cerebrovascular network related to the internal carotid arteries. J Neurosurg 29: 255–260
212. Nishimoto A, Takeuchi S (1972) Moyamoya disease. Abnormal cerebrovascular network in the cerebral basal region. In: Vinken PJ, Bruyn GW (eds): Handbook of clinical neurology, vol 12. North-Holland: Amsterdam, pp 352–383
213. Nishimoto A, Sugiu R, Mannami T (1965) Hemangiomatous malformation of bilateral internal cartodi artery at the base of brain. Brain Nerve (Tokyo) 17: 750–752
214. Nishimoto A, Sugiu R, Takeuchi S (1966) Malformation of Willis. Japanese cases showing a peculiar angiographical pattern. Brain Nerve (Tokyo) 18: 508–513
215. Nishimoto A, Ueta K, Kuyama H, Takemoto M, Arimitsu T, Mizukawa N (1976) Cerebral hemodynamics in moyamoya disease. In: Reports by the research committee on spontaneous occlusion of the circle of Willis. Japanese Ministry of Health and Welfare, Tokyo, pp 76–82
216. Nishimoto A, Mizukawa N, Ueta K, Oube H (1977) Summary of clinical survey. In: Reports by the research committee on spontaneous occlusion of the circle of Willis. Japanese Ministry of Health and Welfare, Tokyo, pp 17–24
217. Nishimoto A, Oube H, Ueta K (1979) Clinical and cerebral blood flow study in moyamoya disease with TIA. Acta Neurol Scand [suppl 72] 60: 434–435
218. Nishimoto A, Ueda K, Oube H (1981) Cooperative study on moyamoya disease in Japan. In: Proceeding of the 10th Japanese conference on surgery of cerebral stroke. Neuron, Tokyo, pp 53–58
219. Nomura T (1965) Occlusion of the circle of Willis with various collateral pathways. Brain Nerve (Tokyo) 17: 33–34
220. Nomura T, Yamagami T, Kawasaki M, Imagawa K, Toda I, Hayashi M, Asai A (1981) On the collateral pathway from the perforating branches to the cortical branches. In: Proceeding of the 10th Japanese conference on surgery of cerebral stroke. Neuron, Tokyo, pp 125–128
221. Nose T (1977) The diagnostic value of radioisotopic investigations in moyamoya. Brain Nerve (Tokyo) 29: 611–619
222. Oda K, Itoyama Y, Shibasaki H, Kuroiwa Y (1978) Moyamoya disease with alexia-agraphia. Neurol Med (Tokyo) 9: 343–348
223. Ogawa A, Sakurai Y, Sato T, Komatsu S, Suzuki J (1981) Continuous measurement of regional cerebral blood flow using Krypton-81m. Brain Nerve (Tokyo) 33: 743–748
224. Ogawa A, Kogure T, Fujiwara, S, Kodama N, Suzuki J, Sakurai Y, Wada N (1981) Regional cerebral blood flow on moyamoya disease: study with ^{133}Xe intravenous injection method. In: Proceeding of the 10th Japanese conference on surgery of cerebral stroke. Neuron, Tokyo, pp 189–194
225. Ogawa Y, Hosoda Y, Matsuyama H (1974) An autopsy case of occlusion of the circle of Willis in a child. Brain Nerve (Tokyo) 26: 483–487

226. Ohashi T, Udea K, Mizukawa N, Nishimoto A, Ikuta F (1975) Autopsy cases of moyamoya disease. Brain Nerve (Tokyo) 27: 1017–1025
227. Oka K, Tanaka K, Sadoshima S, Nakashima T, Nakamura H, Seno S, Nakata K, Maeda R, Hamashima Y, Takahashi M, Ohta G, Kitaoka T, Kotoh K, Sasaki M, Nishihara Y (1979) Intracranial hemorrhage in autopsy cases with occlusion of the circle of Willis. Brain Nerve (Tokyo) 31: 1255–1262
228. Okamoto J, Mukai K, Kashihara M, Ueda S, Matsumoto K (1982) A case of atypical moyamoya disease with a ruptured aneurysm on moyamoya vessel. Neurol Surg (Tokyo) 10: 897–903
229. Okeda (1970) An autopsy case of lung cancer clinically associated with occlusion of distal portion of the bilateral internal carotid arteries and abnormal intracranial vascular networks at the base of the brain. Consideration about pathogenesis of the arterial occlusion and abnormal vascular networks. Adv Neurol Sci (Tokyo) 14: 285–301
230. Okuma A, Oshita H, Funakoshi T, Shikinami A, Yamada H (1980) A case of aneurysm in the cerebral moyamoya vessel: aneurysmal rupture during cerebral angiography and spontaneous regression of the aneurysm. Neurol Surg (Tokyo) 8: 181–185
231. Ohno K, Fujimoto T, Komatsu K, Hiratsuka H, Inaba Y, Kamisasa A, Shibata T (1976) Abnormal intracranial vascular network containing an aneurysm: especially its morphological findings by operating microscope. Brain Nerve 28: 353–364
232. Ohno K, Fujimoto T, Komatsu K, Inaba Y, Ida T (1977) Spontaneous successive occlusion of the circle of Willis with the growth of abnormal vascular networks at the base of the brain. In relation to the pathogenesis of so-called »moyamoya« disease. Brain Nerve (Tokyo) 29: 37–43
233. Onuma T, Yonemitsu T (1981) a case of progressive stenosis of bilateral internal carotid bifurcation with moyamoya vessels which aggravated shortly after head trauma. In: Proceeding of the 10th Japanese conference on surgery of cerebral stroke. Neuron, Tokyo, pp 42–50
234. Osada K (1967) Study of the influence of the autonomic nerve system as regards raising of systemic disease caused by experimental prolonged sensitization. Oto-Rhino-Laryngol Soc Jpn (Tokyo) 70: 987–1006
235. O'Sullivan DJ, Lim GHK, Darveniza P, Coffey GL (1977) Multiple progressive intracranial arterial occlusions (moyamoya disease). J Neurol Neurosurg Psychiatry 40: 853–860
236. Ohta H, Ito Z, Suzuki A, Tominaga S, Uemura K (1981) Regional cerebral blood flow in moyamoya disease evaluated by ^{133}Xe Intracarotid injection method. In: Proceeding of the 10th Japanese conference on surgery of cerebral stroke. Neuron, Tokyo, pp 167–173
237. Otsuki T, Fukawa O, Aihara T (1982) A case of persistent primitive trigeminal artery associated with moyamoya vessels. Jpn J Clin Radiol (Tokyo) 27: 1453–1456
238. Owada K, Hori S, Suzuki J (1979) Results of cervical sympathectomy for cerebral vasospasm following aneurysm rupture. In: Suzuki J (ed) Cerebral aneurysms. Neuron, Tokyo, pp 435–441
239. Padget DH (1948) The development of the cranial arteries in human embryo. Carnegie Inst Wash Publ Contrib Embryol 32: 207–262
240. Pecker J, Simon J, Guy G, Herry JF (1973) Hishimoto's disease. Significance of its angiographic appearances. Neuroradiology 5: 223–230
241. Phelps ME, Hoffman EJ, Huang SC, Kuhl DE (1978) ECAT. A new computerized tomographic imaging system for positron emitting radiopharmaceuticals. J Nucl Med 19: 635–647
242. Picard L, Andre JM, Weber M, Robert J, Tridon P, Arnould G (1972) Stenoses multiples des arteres cerebrales de moyen calibre et reseaux capillaires anormaux (moyamoya). Sem Hop Paris 48: 2049–2055
243. Picard L, Weber M, Andre JM (1973) Le syndrome moya-moya. Rev Electroencephalogr Eur 4: 297–303
244. Picard L, Andre JM, Tridon P (1974) Introduction. Historique du syndrome moyamoya. J Neuroradiol 1: 47–54
245. Picard L, Andre JM, Roland J, Arnould G, Lepoire J, Crouzet G, Djindjian R (1974) Syndrome moyamoya de l'adulte. Formes de passage. J Neuroradiol 1: 69–86

246. Picard L, Floquet J, André JM Montaut J, Salamon G (1974) Syndrome moyamoya. Etude anatomopathologique. J Neuroradiol 1: 113–132
247. Pilz P (1976) Fibromuscular dysplasia and multiple dissecting aneurysms of intracranial arteries. A further cause of moyamoya syndrome. Stroke 7: 393–398
248. Pool JL, Wood EH, Maki Y (1967) On the cases with abnormal vascular network in the cerebral basal region in the United States. In: Kudo T (ed) A disease with abnormal intracranial vascular networks. Spontaneous occlusion of the circle of Willis. Igaku shoin, Tokyo, pp 63–69
249. Poor GY, Gacs GY (1974) The so-called »Moyamoya disease«. J Neurol Neurosurg Psychiatry 37: 370
250. Rajakulasingam K, Carullo LJ, Raimondi AJ (1979) Childhood moyamoya syndrome. Childs Brain 5: 467–475
251. Reilly J, Rivelier E, Compagnon A, Friedmann E, Pham HC, Buit H (1936) Le role du systeme neurovegetatif dans le reactions d'hypersensibile. Ann Med 2: 165–188
252. Ribaric I, Vrankovic D, Janicijevic M, Ivkov M (1976) Multiple progressive intracranial arterial occlusion. Erp Arch Celok Lek 104: 903–911
253. Richman DP, Watts HG, Parsons K, Schmid K, Glimecher, MJ (1977) Familial Moyamoya associated with biochemical abnormalities of connective tissue. Neurology 27: 382
254. Rosengren K (1974) Moyamoya vessels. Collateral arteries of the basal ganglia. Malignant occlusion of the anterior cerebral arteries. Acta Radiol [Diagn] 15: 145–151
255. Rovira M, Torrent O, Ruscalleda J (1975) Etiology of moyamoya disease, acquired or congenital. Acta Radiol [Suppl] 347: 229–240
256. Saito Y (1967) Additional autopsy case report. In: Kudo T (ed) A disease with abnormal intracranial vascular networks. Spontaneous occlusion of the circle of Willis. Igaku shoin, Tokyo, pp 127–128
257. Salyer WR, Salyer DC (1974) The vascular legions of neurofibrimatosis. Angiology 25: 510–519
258. Sano K (1965) Cerebral juxta-basal telangiectasia. Brain Nerve (Tokyo) 17: 748–750
259. Sano K, Kuwabara T, Jimbo M, Saito I (1967) On the cerebral juxta-basal telangiectasia. In: Kudo T (ed) A disease with abnormal intracranial vascular networks. Spontaneous occlusion of the circle of Willis. Igaku shoin, Tokyo, pp 77–83
260. Sato S, Suzuki J (1975) Anatomical mapping of the cerebral nervi vasorum in the human brain. J Neurosurg 13: 559–568
261. Sato T, Sato S, Suzuki J (1979) Correlation with superior cervical sympathetic ganglion and sympathetic nerve innervation of intracranial artery: electron microscopical studies. Brain Nerve (Tokyo) 31: 375–384
262. Schoenberg BS, Mellinger JF, Schoenberg DG (1978) Moyamoya disease in children. South Med J 71: 237–241
263. Seeler RA, Royal JE, Power L, Goldberg H (1978) Moyamoya in children with sickle cell anemia and cerebrovascular occlusion. Pediatrics 93: 808–810
264. Servo A, Puranen M (1978) Moyamoya syndrome as a complication of radiation therapy. J Neurosurg 48: 1026–1029
265. Shellshear JL (1920) The basal arteries of the forebrain and their functional significance. J Anat 55: 27–35
266. Shibuya S, Fukumitsu T, Watanabe T, Yoshida Y, Amo M (1973) Surgical treatment for the case of cerebral arterial rete with intracerebral hermorrhage. Surg Therapy (Osaka) 28: 493–496
267. Shimizu K, Takeuchi K (1955) Hypoplasia of the bilateral internal carotid arteries. The 14th Japan Neurosurgical Society, Wakayama
268. Simon J, Sabouraud O, Guy G, Turpin J (1968) Un cas de maladie de Nishimoto. A propos d'une maladie rare et bilatérale de la carotide interne. Rev Neurol (Paris) 119: 376–383
269. Shirane R, Fujiwara S, Kodama N, Suzuki J, Hiraga H (1981) EEG findings in moyamoya disease. In: Proceeding of the 10th Japanese conference on surgery of cerebral stroke. Neuron, Tokyo, pp 134–139
270. Smith KR, Nelson JS, Dooley JM (1968) Bilateral hypoplasia of the internal carotid arteries. Neurology 18: 1149–1156

271. Sobata E (1980) Efficacy of the cervical sympathectomy in cerebral ischemic patients: measurement of blood flow with a square wave electromagnetic flowmeter and clinical study. Neurol Surg (Tokyo) 8: 739–748
272. Søgaard I, Jørgensen J (1975) Familial occurrence of bilateral intracranial occlusion of the internal carotid arteries (Moya Moya). Acta Neurochir (Wien) 31: 245–252
273. Sonobe M, Takahashi S, Urakawa Y, Nagamine Y, Kodama N, Fukazawa H (1980) »Moyamoya« disease found in identical twins. Neurol Surg (Tokyo) 8: 1183–1188
274. Sonobe M, Takahashi S, Kubota Y, Shirane R (1982) Chronic subdural hematoma developing after EMS for moyamoya disease. Neurol Surg (Tokyo) 10: 857–859
275. Spetzler RF, Roski RA, Kopaniky DR (1980) Alternative superficial temporal artery to middle cerebral artery revascularization procedure. Neurosurgery 7: 484–487
276. Spinivas K, Narayanan M, Gopal S, Jagannathan K (1979) Carotid arterial occlusion in identical twins with moyamoya. Arch Neurol 36: 253–254
277. Stockman JA, Nigro MA, Mishkin MM, Oski FA (1972) Occlusion of large cerebral vessels in sickle cell anemia. N Engl J Med 287: 846
278. Sunder TR, Erwin CW, Dubois PC (1980) Hyperventilation induced abnormalities in the electroencephalogram of children with moyamoya disease. Electroencephalogr Clin Neurophysiol 49: 414–420
279. Sunder TR (1981) Moyamoya disease in a patient with type I glycogenosis. Arch Neurol 38: 251–253
280. Suzuki J (1969) Cerebrovascular moyamoya disease. J Jpn College Angiol (Tokyo) 9:401
281. Suzuki J (1970) Cerebrovascular moyamoya disease. J Jpn College Angiol (Tokyo) 10: 107–113
282. Suzuki J (1971) The disease showing the abnormal vascular network at the base of brain: Transactions of the 18th general assembly of the Japan medical congress. Japan Medical Congress, Tokyo, pp 1263–1266
283. Suzuki J, Kodama N (1971) Cerebrovascular moyamoya disease. Second report: collateral routes to forebrain via ethmoid sinus and superior nasal meatus. Angiology 22: 223–236
284. Suzuki J, Kodama N (1980) Correlation between ventricular hemorrhage and chronic cerebral ischemia in adult moyamoya. In: Pia HW, Langmaid C, Zierski J (eds) Spontaneous intracerebral haematoma, Springer, Berlin Heidelberg New York, pp 145–154
285. Suzuki J, Takaku A (1968) The disease showing the abnormal vascular network at the base of brain particularly found in Japan. III. Etiologic consideration. Diagnosis Treat (Tokyo) 56: 460–472
286. Suzuki J, Takaku A (1968) The disease showing the abnormal vascular network at the base of brain particularly found in Japan. Brain Nerve (Tokyo) 20: 35–40
287. Suzuki J, Takaku A (1969) Cerebrovascular moyamoya disease. Disease showing abnormal net-like vessels in base of brain. Arch Neurol 20: 288–299
288. Suzuki J, Kowada M, Asahi M, Takaku A (1963) The disease showing abnormal vascular network which is thought to be developed collateral pathways. In: Proceedings of the 22nd Meeting of the Japan Neurosurgical Society
289. Suzuki J, Kowada M, Asahi M, Takaku A (1965) Diseases showing the »fibrille« like vessels at the base of brain. Frequently found in Japan. Brain Nerve (Tokyo) 17: 767–776
290. Suzuki J, Takaku A, Asahi M (1966) The disease showing the abnormal vascular network at the base of brain, particularly found in Japan. II. A following-up study. Brain Nerve (Tokyo) 18: 897–908
291. Suzuki J, Takaku A, Asahi M (1967) Etiological consideration of moyamoya disease. In: Kudo T (ed) A disease with abnormal intracranial vascular networks. Spontaneous occlusion of the circle of Willis. Igaku shoin, Tokyo, pp 73–75
292. Suzuki J, Takaku A, Fukazawa H (1967) Cerebrovascular »Moyamoya« disease among the Japanese, on study of an autopsy case. In: Kudo T (ed) A disease with abnormal intracranial vascular networks. Spontaneous occlusion of the circle of Willis. Igaku shoin, Tokyo, pp 93–98
293. Suzuki J, Kodama N, Takaku A (1970) Collateral passway via »Ethmoidal moyamoya« in cerebrovascular »Moyamoya« disease, disease showing abnormal net-like vessels in base of brain. Brain Nerve (Tokyo) 22: 417–424

294. Suzuki J, Takaku A, Kodama N, Satoh S (1975) An attempt to treat cerebrovascular ›Moyamoya‹ disease in children. Childs Brain 1: 193–206
295. Suzuki J, Iwabuchi T, Hori S (1975) Cervical sympathectomy for cerebral vasospasm after aneurysm rupture. Neurol Med Chir (Tokyo) 15(I): 41–50
296. Suzuki J, Kodama N, Mineura K (1976) Mechanism of symptomatic occurrence in cerebrovascular moyamoya disease. Brain Nerve (Tokyo) 28: 459–470
297. Suzuki J, Kodama N, Fujiwara S (1978) CT findings in moyamoya disease. In: Reports by the research committee on spontaneous occlusion of the circle of Willis. Japanese Ministry of Health and Welfare, Tokyo, pp 44–48
298. Suzuki J, Kodama N, Fujiwara S (1979) Pathological study on autopsy cases of moyamoya disease. In: Reports by the research committee on spontaneous occlusion of the circle of Willis. Japanese Ministry of Health and Welfare, Tokyo, pp 105–109
299. Suzuki J, Kodama N, Fujiwara S, Kasai N, Yonemitsu T (1981) The experimental study on causal genesis of moyamoya disease. Correlation with immunological reaction and sympathetic nerve influence for vascular change. In: Reports by the research committee on spontaneous occlusion of the circle of Willis. Japanese Ministry of Health and Welfare, Tokyo, pp 21–34
300. Takahashi M (1980) Magnification angiography in moyamoya disease. New observations on collateral vessels. Radiology 136: 379–386
301. Takahashi M, Miyauchi T, Kowada M (1980) Computed tomography of moyamoya disease. Occluded arteries and collateral vessels as important diagnostic signs. Radiology 134: 671–676
302. Takahashi M, Saito Y, Konno K (1980) Intraventricular hemorrhage in childhood moyamoya disease. Case report. Comput Assist Tomogr 4: 117–120
303. Takahashi S, Kutsuzawa T, Takahashi S (1967) Studies on cerebral hemodynamics. In: Kudo T (ed) A disease with abnormal intracranial vascular networks. Spontaneous occlusion of the circle of Willis. Igaku shoin, Tokyo, pp 35–37
304. Takaku A (1966) Cerebral angiography in mentally retarded children. 1st report. Clin Neurol (Tokyo) 6: 379–385
305. Takamura H, Yada K, Tsuru M (1966) Nine cases showing the abnormal vascular network at the base of the brain. Brain Nerve (Tokyo) 18: 515–518
306. Takebe Y, Haneda S, Mita R (1979) Clinical pictures and EEG findings of the children with cerebrovascular »moyamoya« disease. Clin Encephaloelectrogr (Tokyo) 21: 694–699
307. Takemoto M, Motoki M, Yoshioka J, Miyake I, Baba Y, Doi A (1981) Follow-up study of moyamoya disease with Tc-RBCs vascular imaging. In: Proceeding of the 10th Japanese conference on surgery of cerebral stroke. Neuron, Tokyo, pp 301–305
308. Takeuchi K (1967) Clinical cases in childhood. In: Kudo T (ed) A disease with abnormal intracranial vascular networks. Spontaneous occlusion of the circle of Willis. Igaku shoin Tokyo, pp 59–62
309. Takeuchi K (1978) Moyamoya phenomenon and moyamoya disease. Brain Nerve (Tokyo) 30: 1183–1191
310. Takeuchi S (1967) Studies on Japanese cases with abnormal vascular network at the base of the brain in cerebral angiography: Part I. Clinical Invest Okayama Igakkai Zasshi (Okayama) 79: 311–336
311. Takeuchi S (1967) Studies on Japanese cases with abnormal vascular network at the base of the brain in cerebral angiography: Part II. Animal experiment on its pathogenesis. Okayama Igakkai Zasshi (Okayama) 79: 337–345
312. Takeuchi K, Akai K (1972) Moymoya phenomenon and moyamoya disease. Acta Neurol Scand [suppl 72] 60: 446–447
313. Takeuchi K, Kobayashi S (1965) Child's case showing the occlusion of arteries at the base of the brain. Brain Nerve (Tokyo) 17: 779–780
314. Takeuchi K, Shimizu K (1957) Hypoplasia of the bilateral internal carotid arteries. Brain Nerve (Tokyo) 9: 37–43
315. Takeuchi K, Hara M, Yokota H, Okada J, Akai K (1981) Factors influencing the development of moyamoya phenomenon. In: Proceeding of the 10th Japanese conference on surgery of cerebral stroke. Neuron, Tokyo, pp 31–35

316. Takeuchi S, Kobayashi K, Tsuchida T, Ishii R, Tanaka R, Ito J (1981) Regional cerebral blood flow in moyamoya disease: study of epicerebral microcirculation by fluorescein angiography. In: Proceeding of the 10th Japanese conference on surgery of cerebral stroke. Neuron, Tokyo, pp 199–204
317. Takeyama E, Matsumori K, Sugimori T, Kagawa M, Fukuyama Y (1976) A case of the anterior choroidal artery aneurysm combined with the abnormal intracranial vascular network. Neurol Surg (Tokyo) 4: 1075–1079
318. Taki W, Yonekawa Y, Matsuda I, Moritake K, Yamagata S, Handa H (1979) STA-MCA bypass for so-called moyamoya disease. In: Proceeding of the 8th Japanese conference on surgery of cerebral stroke. Neuron, Tokyo, pp 269–273
319. Tamaki N, Matsuda T (1970) Cerebral rete mirabile anastmoses. Brain Nerve (Tokyo) 22: 405–412
320. Tanaka K, Oka K (1978) Autopsy cases of occlusion of circle of Willis. In: Reports by the research committee on spontaneous occlusion of the circle of Willis. Japanese Ministry of Health and Welfare, Tokyo, pp 103–107
321. Tanaka K, Oka K (1979) Occlusion of circle of Willis with intracerebral hemorrhage. In: Reports by the research committee on spontaneous occlusion of the circle of Willis. Japanese Ministry of Health and Welfare, Tokyo, pp 100–104
322. Tanaka K, Yamashita M (1981) Intracranial vascular lesions of occlusion of circle of Willis. In: Reports by the research committee on spontaneous occlusion of the circle of Willis. Japanese Ministry of Health and Welfare, Tokyo, pp 134–138
323. Tanaka K, Yamashita M (1981) Pathology of moyamoya disease. In: Proceeding of the 10th Japanese conference on surgery of cerebral stroke. Neuron, Tokyo, pp 159–164
324. Tanaka N, Okamoto K, Naoe S (1975) Autopsy cases of muco-cutaneous lymphnode syndrome, in relation to arteritis in infants. Pediatrics Jpn (Tokyo) 16: 886–895
325. Tanaka Y, Takeuchi K, Ogashiwa M, Akai K, Omata K (1978) Moyamoya phenomenon combined with cerebral aneurysm. Brain Nerve (Tokyo) 30: 687–695
326. Taveras JM (1969) Multiple progressive intracranial arterial occlusions. A syndrome of children and young adults. AJR 106: 235–268
327. Tazaki Y, Furuhashi N, Kanda T, Kobayashi S, Hayakawa I, Hayashi H (1980) Cerebral circulation in occlusion of the circle of Willis. In: Reports by the research committee on spontaneous occlusion of the circle of Willis. Japanese Ministry of Health and Welfare, Tokyo, pp 56–61
328. Tazaki Y, Sakai F, Kitai N, Asakura H (1982) Regional cerebral blood flow in occlusion of the circle of Willis. In: Reports by the research committee on spontaneous occlusion of the circle of Willis. Japanese Ministry of Health and Welfare, Tokyo, pp 98–104
329. Tochio H, Kawasaki M, Imagawa K, Toda I, Hayashi M, Asai A, Nomura T (1978) A comparative study of the clinical features, computed tomography, and electroencephalographic examination of moyamoya disease. Prog Comput Tomogr (Tokyo) 1: 257–271
330. Tomsick TA, Lukin RR, Chambers AA, Benton C (1976) Neurofibromatosis and intracranial arterial occlusive disease. Neuroradiology 11: 229
331. Tsubokawa T, Kikuchi M, Asano S, Itoh H, Urabe M (1964) Surgical treatment for intracranial thrombosis. Case report of »Durapexia«. Neurol Med Chir (Tokyo) 6(I): 428–429
332. Tsubokawa T, Miyanaga M, Fukuda A (1966) Cerebral arterial occlusive disease in childhood and abnormal intracranial vascular networks. Brain Nerve (Tokyo) 18: 539–547
333. Tsuchimoto S, Karasawa J, Kikuchi H, Takahashi N, Iwayama K (1981) Changes in somatosensory evoked potentials of children with »moyamoya« disease. In: Proceeding of the 10th Japanese conference of surgery of cerebral stroke. Neuron, Tokyo, pp 340–344
334. Uemura K, Yamaguchi K, Kojima S, Sakurai Y, Ito Z, Kawakami H, Kutsuzawa T (1975) Regional cerebral blood flow on cerebrovascular »moyamoya« disease: Study by ^{133}Xe clearance method and cerebral angiography. Brain Nerve (Tokyo) 27: 385–393
335. Uemura K, Takahashi A, Kawada Y, Kutsuzawa T, Tominaga S (1980) Regional cerebral blood flow on moyamoya disease. In: Reports by the research committee on spontaneous occlusion of the circle of Willis. Japanese Ministry of Health and Welfare, Tokyo, pp 62–64

336. Umezu R, Fujiu M, Abe (1973) Two cases of von Recklinghausen's disease with juxtabasal telangiectasia. Clin Neurol (Tokyo) 13: 11–16
337. Vila F, Izquierdo JM, Dierssen G, Esparza J (1973) Enfermedad de moyamoya. A propósito de un caso del adulto. Rev Clin Esp 130: 539–542
338. Vinas JMP, Soriano JR, Cordoba AP, Lavin AC, Vargas LM (1973) Étude neuroradiologique d'un cas de syndrome »crane en feuille de tréfle«. Associé avec le syndrome de »moyamoya«. Bordeaux Méd 11: 1635–1641
339. Vuia O, Alexianu M, Gabor S (1970) Hypoplasia and obstruction of the circle of Willis in a case of atypical cerebral hemorrhage and its relationship to Nishimoto's disease. Neurology 20: 361–367
340. Wada T, Aoki Y (1977) Electroencephalographic findings in cerebrovascular moyamoya disease. II. Follow-up study. In: Reports by the research committee on spontaneous occlusion of the circle of Willis. Japanese Ministry of Health and Welfare, Tokyo, pp 52–55
341. Watanabe S, Atsumi H, Okada S, Nishio T (1966) A case showing abnormal vascular network at the unilateral carotisgabel. Brain Nerve (Tokyo) 18: 553–573
342. Weidner W, Hanafee W, Markham CH (1965) Intracranial collateral circulation via leptomeningeal and rete mirabile anastomoses. Neurology 15: 39–48
343. Ximin I, Xuzhong R, Zhuan C, Burun Y, Shangpu H, Yunhe G (1980) Moyamoya disease caused by leptospiral cerebral arteritis. Chinese Med J 93: 599–604
344. Yamada F, Fukuda S, Kawamoto S, Kudo T (1981) Spontaneous occlusion of the circle of Willis: magnification angiographical study of miliary aneurysm as the cause of hemorrhage and its incidence in juvenile and adult groups. In: Proceedings of the 10th Japanese conference on surgery of cerebral stroke. Neuron, Tokyo, pp 94–98
345. Yamada H, Nakamura S, Kageyama N (1980) Moyamoya disease in monovular twins. Case report. J Neurosurg 53: 109–112
346. Yamaguchi T, Tashiro M, Minematsu K, Kitamura K (1980) Summary of Japanese survey of occlusion of the circle of Willis. In: Reports by the research committee on spontaneous occlusion of the circle of Willis. Japanese Ministry of Health and Welfare, Tokyo, pp 13–22
347. Yamaguchi Y (1955) Reilly's phenomenon. Le rule du systéme neurovégétatif dans les réactions d'hypersensibilité. Saishin Igaku (Osaka) 10: 366–374
348. Yamamoto T, Ban S, Inutsuka N, Ogata M, Kato M, Ando K (1974) Electroencephalographic study of intracranial abnormal vascular network. Clin Electroencephalogr (Osaka) 16: 50–54
349. Yasargil MG, Yonekawa Y, Denton I, Piroth D, Benes I (1974) Experimental intracranial transplantation of autogenic omentum majas. J Neurosurg 40: 213–217
350. Yashon D, Johnson AB, Jane JA (1964) Bilateral internal carotid artery occlusion secondary to closed head injuries. J Neurol Neurosurg Psychiatry 27: 547–552
351. Yonekawa Y, Yasargil MG (1977) Brain vascularization by transplanted omentum. A possible treatment of cerebral ischemia. Neurosurgery 1: 256–259
352. Yonekawa Y, Handa H (1980) Surgical treatment of occlusive cerebrovascular diseases. Brain Nerve (Tokyo) 32: 239–255
353. Yonemitsu T, Fujiwara S, Suzuki J (1984) The experimental study on causal genesis of Moyamoya disease — Immunohistochemical investigation —. J Jpn Coll Angiol (Tokyo) 24(7): 537–547
354. Yoshii N, Kudo T (1967) EEG findings of occlusion of the circle of Willis. In: Kudo T (ed) A disease with abnormal intracranial vascular networks. Spontaneous occlusion of the circle of Willis. Igaku shoin, Tokyo, pp 69–72
355. Yoshii N, Kudo T (1968) Electroencephalographical study on occlusion of the Willis arterial ring. Clin Neurol (Tokyo) 8: 301–309
356. Yoshii N, Samejima H, Mizokami T, Ushikubo Y, Kuramitsu T, Sato T, Fukuda A, Yamada F (1981) Long term follow-up study of »moyamoya disease« (Occlusion of circle of Willis) with drug therapy. In: Proceeding of the 10th Japanese conference on surgery of cerebral stroke. Neuron, Tokyo, pp 12–15
357. Yoshii Y (1977) Follow-up study of the »moyamoya«. Brain Nerve (Tokyo) 29: 421–424
358. Yoshii Y (1977) Follow-up study of the »moyamoya«. Brain Nerve (Tokyo) 29: 505–510

359. Zlotnik ZI, Kuznetsov VF, Kastritskaya ZM, Bezzubik SD (1978) Moyamoya disease. Zh Vopr Neirokhir 2: 41–46
360. Zülch KJ, Dreesbach HA, Eschbach O (1974) Occlusion of the middle cerebral artery with the formation of an abnormal arterial collateral system — moyamoya type — 23 months later. Neuroradiology 7: 19–24
361. Zeek PM (1953) Periarteritis nodosa and other forms of necrotizing angitis. N Engl J Med 248: 764–772

Subject Index

GPSR Compliance

The European Union's (EU) General Product Safety Regulation (GPSR) is a set of rules that requires consumer products to be safe and our obligations to ensure this.

If you have any concerns about our products, you can contact us on ProductSafety@springernature.com

In case Publisher is established outside the EU, the EU authorized representative is:

Springer Nature Customer Service Center GmbH
Europaplatz 3
69115 Heidelberg, Germany

Batch number: 10704763

Printed by Printforce, the Netherlands